The
ULTIMATE
FERTILITY
COOKBOOK
For Couples

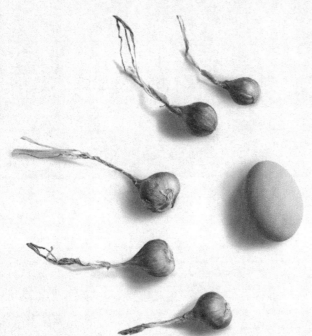

100 Curated Fun, Delicious, and
Healthy Recipes to Improve Fertility

OLIVIA PHILLIPS

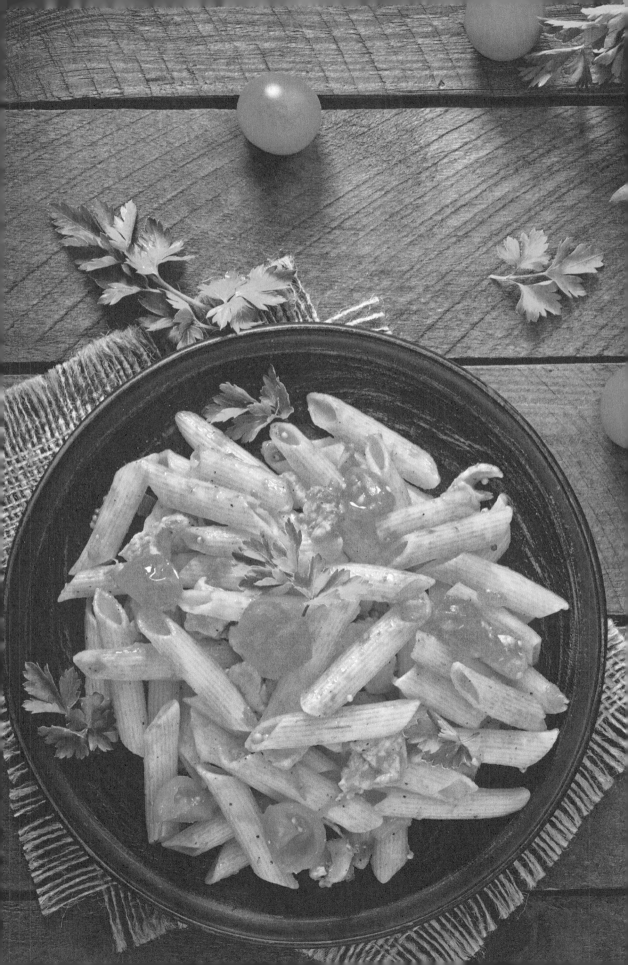

Table of Contents

Introduction

Fertility refers to both men and women's reproductive health and their abilities to create a child. For a woman, her reproductive system, which includes the uterus, ovaries, and other organs, relies on certain vitamins and nutrients to function properly. And fertility health is for more than just women. Men rely on certain vitamins and nutrients for their reproductive system to work in tip-top shape too.

When it comes to healthy reproductive systems, a fetus is created when a sperm fertilizes an egg. That fetus latches to the wall of the uterus where it should grow for roughly nine months before being born into the world. While pregnant, everything the mother eats or ingests is also ingested by the baby. That is why a fertility diet and other healthy eating habits are important not only when you are trying to conceive, but throughout all nine months of pregnancy as well. Certain foods are even beneficial for specific organ development within the future child. You can also eat specific foods to assist in specific areas of reproduction. For example, Spinach which is rich in vitamin A and folate, is specifically useful for egg health and the production of strong eggs in a woman's body.

The process of conceiving a child is easier for some than others, but one of the simplest ways to give yourself a fertility boost is through nutrition. When you eat the right foods, you increase your chances of conceiving naturally and of having a successful IVF treatment.

Most people turn to fertility diets as the first stop along their healthy reproductive journey. You have likely opened this book because you are interested in having a child, or are in the midst of trying to expand your family, and you want to make sure both your body and the future child's body are as healthy as possible. Perhaps you've turned to fertility diets because there is a history of fertility related issues in you or your partner's family and you want to combat those issues naturally. No matter why you are interested in following a fertility diet, you will find the answers and recipes that you seek within these pages. Before beginning any new diet, or beginning your journey to parenthood, make sure to consult your physician or OB GYN. They will have information on your specific health needs that can assist you in how you rely on this cookbook. Consult a doctor prior to using any of the nutritional supplements listed in this book as well.

This cookbook is packed with 100 recipes that will boost both men and women's fertility. Unlike other cookbooks that will keep you cooking in the kitchen for hours, these recipes are focused on realistic cooking and utilizing ingredients you likely already have in your fridge. Follow along for fun and tasty recipes for breakfast, lunch, dinner, dessert, snacks, and drinks. They are so good, your dinner guests won't even realize they are getting a fertility boost from dining with you. Many of these recipes are also great to make with your partner on a fun 'date-night' in.

These recipes include some of the traditional fertility power-house foods like oysters and liver that most people assume take lots of skill to cook, but these recipes will break down the steps so that anyone can enjoy a meal that includes the seemingly complicated ingredients of oysters and liver. Don't be fooled, these proteins are healthy and delicious.

Before diving into the recipes, we will cover the basics of fertility diets, what affects fertility, and what foods to focus on specifically whether you are creating meals from this book or experimenting on your own. The recipes include dishes for breakfast, lunch, dinner, dessert, snacks and sides, and beverages. With help from this guide, you can include fertility friendly foods in every meal of your day. To learn how, read on!

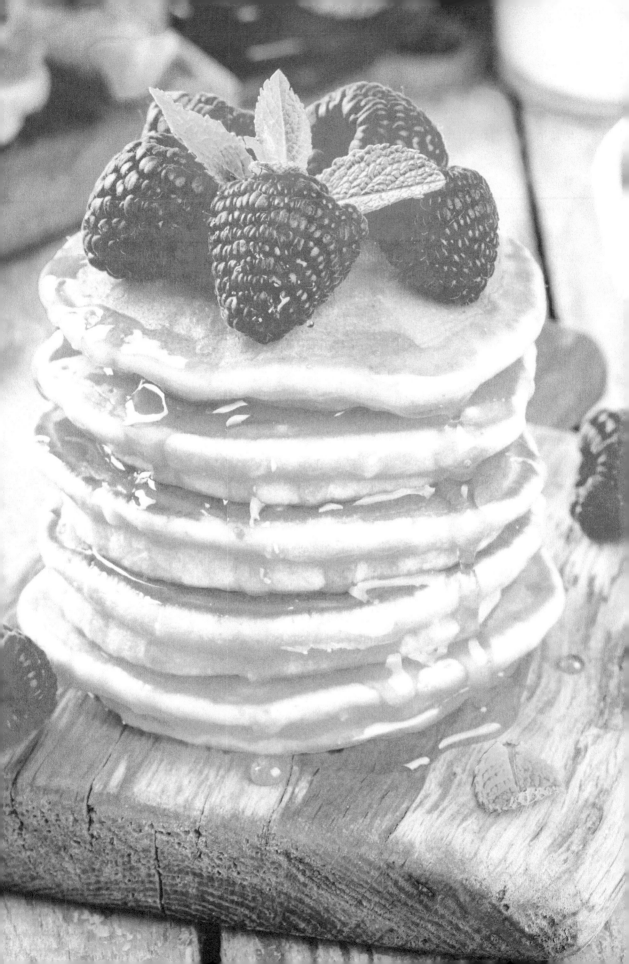

CHAPTER ONE

Understanding the Basics of Fertility

Improving your fertility sounds like a daunting task, but it isn't really so hard. Before you can start cooking up a storm, we are going to cover the fertility basics. What affects fertility? What to eat in general? And how the vitamins and nutrients present in some of our favorite foods are doing us unexpected favors.

In general, women are born with 300,000 eggs. They never create anymore. Men, on the other hand, produce sperm every few months for their entire lives. Not everyone is lucky enough to have healthy sperm and eggs, or well functioning reproductive systems. Diet is the first change that you can make towards becoming more fertile. It is also the easiest, as the remaining options include IVF, surrogacy, and other medical procedures.

During a healthy conception, a sperm will penetrate an egg that has been released from the ovaries in a process known as fertilization. Once fertilized, the egg will implant on the wall of the uterus and grow there for roughly 40 weeks. During the development of the fetus, it intakes everything the mother intakes. It develops organs, skin, and bones, so that after 40 weeks, it is born into this world as a human child.

However, not all conceptions are successful. Some men can have weak sperm. Some women can have unhealthy eggs. There can be nutrient deficiencies that do not allow the egg to attach to the wall of the uterus. And, once a pregnancy is confirmed, it is still important to eat fertility boosting foods so that the fetus develops properly. There are several other things that can affect fertility, both positively and negatively that we will address in the next section.

What Affects Fertility

The two most basic factors on a person's fertility are diet and exercise. Healthier people have a better chance of being fertile. Especially in men, being overweight can make it more difficult to produce healthy sperm and maintain healthy hormone levels. According to Cedars Sinai, "30% of infertility cases are solely due to problems with sperm production," (Cedars-Sinai, 2017). For this reason, we start by examining diet and exercise as effects on fertility. This doesn't mean you have to be a powerlifter or marathon runner to have a child, but a generally healthy diet and regular, light exercise will give you a reproductive head start.

For women, common medical problems like Polycystic Ovary Syndrome (PCOS) and Endometriosis can also negatively impact fertility. In some cases, they can restrict a woman from having children at all. Women with PCOS experience prolonged or irregular menstrual cycles, they have an increased amount of male hormones in their bodies, and their ovaries suffer from collecting pockets of fluid. Women with Endometriosis have tissue growing on the outside of their uterus when it should be growing on the inside of their uterus. This disease can create problems for women trying to conceive because the tissue is essential for the egg to latch to the wall of the uterus.

Finally, age for both genders can ultimately be a barrier to conceiving. Women tend to go through menopause around the age of 45 to 55. After menopause, women are no longer fertile. And, even though men continue to produce sperm throughout their lifetime, the health and vitality of that sperm does decrease as men age.

Vitamins and Other Ways to Nourish Your Body

Along with larger scale dietary changes, it can be important to implement vitamins and supplements into your diet when you first begin your fertility journey. Even something as simple as a multivitamin can increase your health dramatically. There are basic fertility and prenatal vitamins available online and in brick and mortar stores that can be a good place to start. Anything that increases your vitamin E, vitamin D, vitamin B12, and iron will affect your fertility.

Other natural supplements like bee pollen and collagen powder are great ways to boost fertility as well.

Outside of nutrition, those trying to get pregnant should reduce their stress levels through mindfulness, yoga, or therapy. And, try to stay active. Exercise and reduced stress will not only make you feel better mentally, but they will have physical effects as well, like increased fertility.

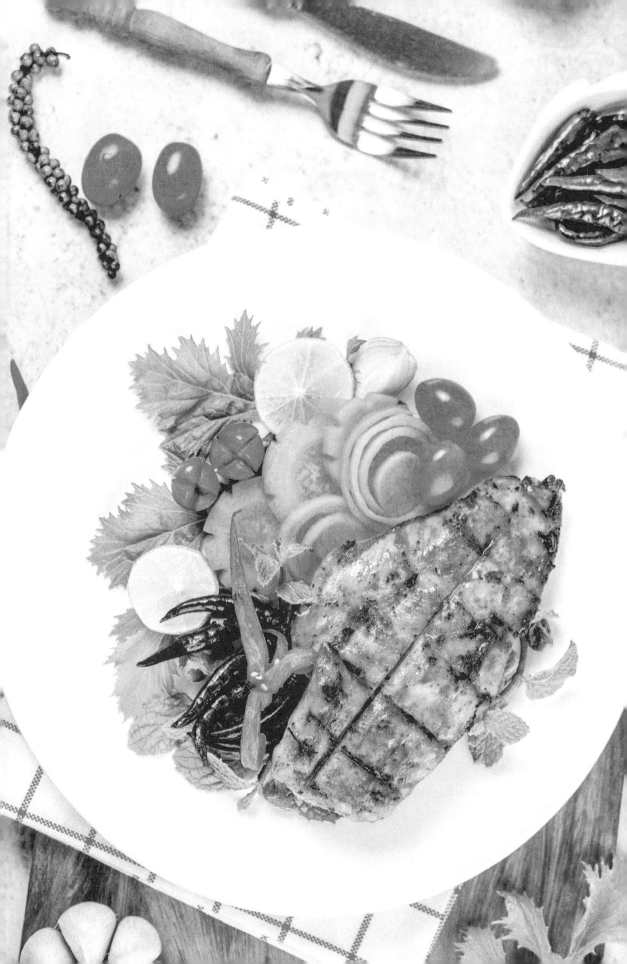

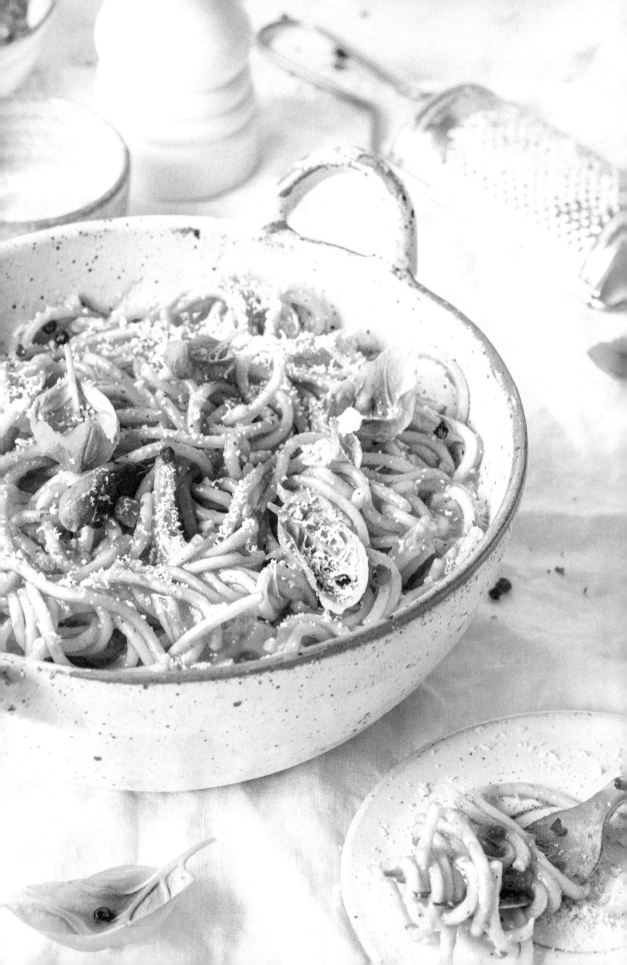

CHAPTER TWO

The Science Behind the Fertility Diet

The fertility diet gives couples the best odds for conceiving easily and naturally. It is always the best place to start, because it is an easy lifestyle change, relatively inexpensive, and doesn't involve trips to the doctor. The diet increases fertility health based on the vitamins and nutrients found in foods that correlate to the biological processes of the reproductive system.

Keep in mind that it takes 70 to 90 days for sperm and egg to develop. So, even when following this diet, you won't see results for 2 to 3 months.

Overall the foods that you eat on a fertility diet should reduce inflammation. Inflammation can be caused by excessive carbohydrates from sugars and fibers. Certain plant toxins, like phytoestrogen, can also cause inflammation. The ingredients in your diet should lean towards a high-fat and low-carb make up in order to reduce as much inflammation as possible. Generally, women with higher levels of inflammation have more trouble conceiving. Higher levels of cholesterol are also key to a well balanced fertility diet. Cholesterol, while typically given a bad reputation, is important for healthy hormone balancing and progesterone creation. "A team of Harvard researchers in 2007, the "Fertility Diet" study— found women with ovulatory infertility who followed this eating pattern had a 66% lower risk of ovulatory infertility and a 27% reduced risk of infertility from other causes than women who didn't follow the diet closely," (Eat Right, 2020).

Foods to Eat and Foods to Avoid for Him and Her

All of the recipes you will find in the remaining sections will adhere to these ingredients list, as well as including a few other healthy options. Remember that the food choices you make are important for both male and female fertility. For best results, both soon-to-be parents should incorporate as many of these fertility boosting foods into their diets as possible. And, not everything overlaps, so what is fertility boosting for men may not be fertility boosting for women.

Each of these ingredients will improve your reproductive health in different ways. For example, onions can improve the quality of men's sperm, but they don't have any particular effects in women. Meanwhile, Brazil nuts are fantastic for women's ovulatory process and the creation of strong eggs. They are a great source of plant-based protein for men, but have fewer reproductive benefits.

Foods to Eat (Her)

- Steak
- Liver
- Salmon
- Eggs
- Sardines
- Pork Belly
- Butter
- Full Fat Dairy
- Whole Milk
- Whole Fat Yogurt
- Cheese
- Asparagus
- Leafy Greens
- Spinach
- Kale
- Pomegranates
- Walnuts
- Brazil Nuts
- Beans
- Pumpkin
- Sweet Potato
- Chickpeas
- Sunflower Seeds
- Citrus Fruits

- Oranges
- Lemon
- Grapefruit
- Cooked Tomatoes
- Avocado
- Oysters
- Cinnamon
- Beets

Foods to Eat (Him)

- Steak
- Liver
- Salmon
- Eggs
- Sardines
- Pork Belly
- Butter
- Full Fat Dairy
- Whole Milk
- Whole Fat Yogurt
- Cheese
- Asparagus
- Leafy Greens
- Spinach
- Kale
- Pomegranates
- Walnuts
- Beans
- Pumpkin
- Sweet Potato
- Chickpeas

- Sunflower Seeds
- Citrus Fruits
- Oranges
- Lemon
- Grapefruit
- Cooked Tomatoes
- Avocado
- Oysters
- Cinnamon
- Beets
- Onions

Foods to Avoid

- Soy
- Alcohol
- Caffeine
- Simple Sugars
- Carbohydrates
- High glycemic index fruits

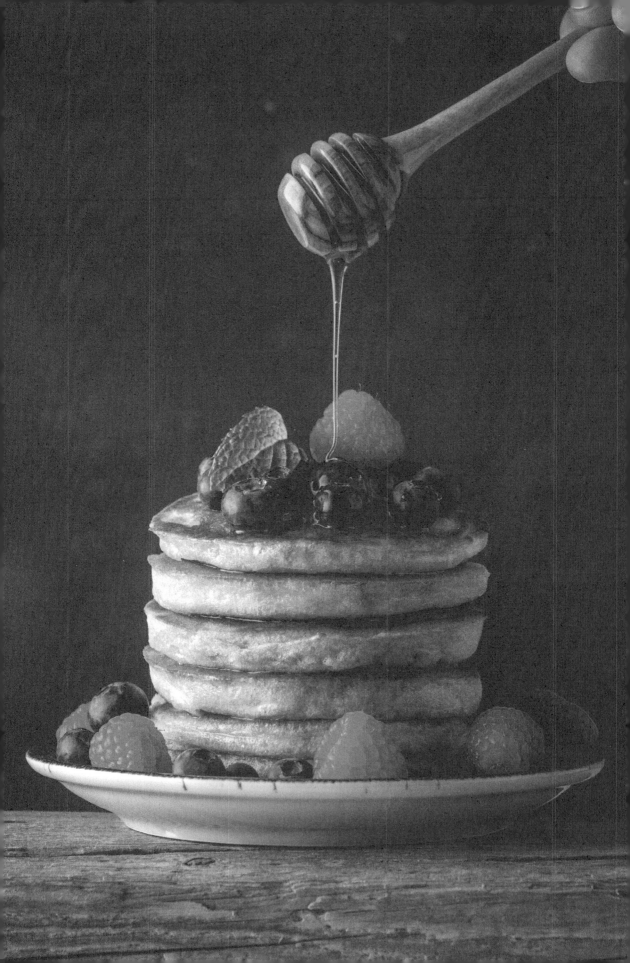

CHAPTER THREE

Breakfast

The benefits of a fertility diet don't have to wait until lunch or dinner. We've compiled several breakfast recipes that include the key fertility friendly foods like avocados, eggs, liver, spinach, and pomegranates. Many of these recipes can be cooked quickly on a weekday morning, others are fun to make for longer amounts of time on the weekends with your partner. Make it a breakfast date! No matter how you choose to enjoy these dishes, one thing is for sure, they will build an effective fertility diet that balances your hormones and boosts fertility in both men and women. Taste test some of my particular favorites, like the smoked salmon eggs benedict, the banana oat muffins, and the quiche. And, don't stop the fertility diet just because you've received a positive pregnancy test. Keep eating these delicious meals all throughout your pregnancy to keep you and your baby healthy.

For best results, you'll want to make sure you have all the right tools in the kitchen. The most common tools required in these recipes include good knives for chopping vegetables, a cutting board, pots and pans, a toaster, and parchment paper.

Smoked Salmon Eggs Benedict

Salmon is a great source of protein and omega-3 fatty acids for both men and women trying to conceive. Those extra omegas can result in healthier, stronger sperm, and they will help embryo development later on. Salmon recipes are common for dinners, but you can enjoy this fish anytime of day. It makes for a great twist on the classic eggs benedict, which is a recipe that is already off to a great start in the fertility category. Eggs, butter, and other fats present in this recipe will work with the salmon to foster fertility. What's even better? You can buy smoked salmon directly from the grocery store. It doesn't require any additional cooking, so breakfast can be on the table faster.

Time: 1 hour
Serving Size: 2
Prep Time: 45 minutes
Cook Time: 15 minutes
Nutritional Facts/Info:
668 calories, 25 g fat, 79 g protein, 27 g carbohydrates, and 3 g sugar

Ingredients:

- 4 slices smoked salmon
- 4 eggs
- 4 whole grain english muffins
- ½ cup butter
- 1 tbsp lemon juice
- 4 egg yolks
- 2 tbsp cold water
- 1 tsp paprika

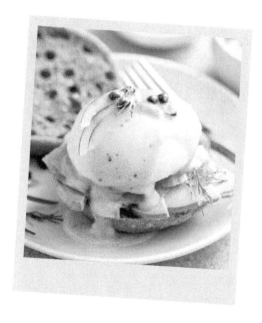

1. Begin by assembling the hollandaise sauce. Place a cup of water in a small pot on the stove and turn to low heat. Set a heat-safe bowl on top of the pot to create a double boiler.

2. Place a second pot of water on the stove top, add salt, and turn the burner to high heat. Wait for this pot to come to a rolling boil.

3. In a separate bowl, crack four eggs separating the yolks. The best way to extract the yolk is by cracking the egg in the center and transferring the yolk between the two shell halves several times. Each time the yolk transfers to a new side of the egg, it will shed more of the egg white until it has fully separated. Whisk the four egg yolks together.

4. Stir the lemon juice into the whisked egg yolks.

5. Add the yolk and lemon juice mixture to the double boiler, stir constantly so the eggs don't curdle.

6. Slowly pour the melted butter into the yolk and lemon juice mixture. Continue to stir until the whole mixture has thickened. If the mixture begins to separate at any point, remove from the heat and add the 2 tbsp of cold water. Continue to stir the sauce as you finish cooking the remainder of the meal.

7. Add the English muffins to a toaster or oven broiler to give them a nice crunch.

8. In the second pot, stir the boiling water with a heat-safe spoon until a whirl pool is created. Crack an egg into the swirling water and continue to stir as the egg cooks. This will poach the egg and should result in a ball shape. Cook each egg for 3–5 minutes depending on your desired egg-firmness.

9. Remove the cooked eggs from the water and set aside.

10. To assemble, begin by placing an English muffin on the plate. Top with a slice of smoked salmon, one poached egg, and a ladle of hollandaise sauce. Sprinkle paprika over the whole plate and enjoy hot!

Sweet Oatmeal

Oatmeal is fantastic for improving fertility because of its high levels of fiber and low glycemic index. This combination makes oatmeal the perfect carb to enjoy while trying to conceive, because it won't raise your blood sugar levels the way a piece of toast might. Adding ingredients like cinnamon, pomegranate, and walnuts to your breakfast oatmeal will make this dish a fertility power house!

And, if you prefer overnight oats to those heated in the microwave, feel free to adjust this recipe by adding the oats and the same measurement of milk or water to the fridge the previous evening.

Time: 10 minutes
Serving Size: 1
Prep Time: 7 minutes
Cook Time: 3 minutes
Nutritional Facts/Info:
309 calories, 26 g fat, 11 g protein, 26 g carbohydrates, 3 g sugar

Ingredients:

- ½ cup steel cut oats
- 1 cup of water (or follow oatmeal package instructions)
- 2 tsp cinnamon
- ¼ cup pomegranate seeds
- ¼ chopped walnuts

1. In a microwave safe bowl, mix the steel cut oats and water.
2. Microwave for 2 minutes, stir the mixture, add the cinnamon, and microwave for an additional minute.
3. Allow the bowl to cool before adding the pomegranate seeds and chopped walnuts.
4. Serve hot!

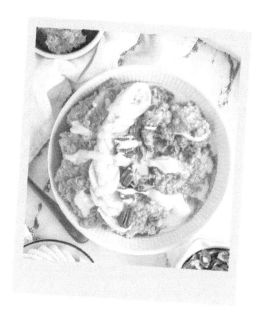

Avocado and Egg Toast

Eggs, known for their high protein content, are great, natural ways to increase your fertility. Avocados are also one of the best vegetables to include in your fertility diet. You can use any type of bread you'd like for this recipe, including gluten free and keto breads to reduce the amount of carbohydrates in your diet.

Time: 15 minutes

Serving Size: 1 serving

Prep Time: 5 minutes

Cook Time: 10 minutes

Nutritional Facts/Info:

605 calories, 49 g fat, 18 g protein, 29 g carbohydrates, 3 g sugar

Ingredients:

- 1 avocado
- 2 eggs
- 2 slices bread
- ½ tbsp butter
- 1 tsp red pepper flakes
- 1 tsp garlic powder
- Salt and pepper

Directions:

1. Place a skillet on a burner set to medium heat. Add the pad of butter and allow to melt.
2. While the butter is melting, cut your avocado in half and remove the skins. Slice lengthwise so you have ten or more thin slices of avocado. Set aside.

3. Once heated, crack two eggs into the skillet. Season the eggs to your taste with garlic powder, salt, and pepper. Cook the eggs on this side for roughly four minutes.

4. While the eggs cook, place two slices of bread in a toaster or under the oven broiler.

5. Flip the eggs until the whites are firm, being careful not to break the yolk.

6. Cook on the opposite side for two additional minutes.

7. Place the toasted bread on a plate, top with the sliced avocado.

8. Remove the over medium eggs from the pan and layer on top of the avocado toast.

9. Season the dish with red pepper flakes and enjoy warm!

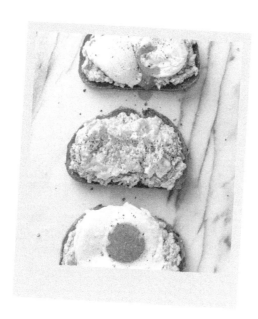

Breakfast Burrito

Breakfast burritos are great sources of protein, and can be packed full of fertility friendly ingredients. They are also a fun breakfast food for partners to cook together. You can even incorporate breakfast burritos into your meal prepping by freezing them for a few days at a time.

In this recipe, we recommend using black beans for an added source of protein. Keep an eye out for BPAs if you use canned beans, as those can have harmful effects to your body. To avoid BPAs, purchase the dried lentils that need to be soaked in water overnight prior to cooking.

Time: 15 minutes

Serving Size: 2 burritos

Prep Time: 5 minutes

Cook Time: 10 minutes

Nutritional Facts/Info:

554 calories, 30 g fat, 26 g protein, 50 g carbohydrates, 4 g sugar

Ingredients:

- 2 whole-grain tortillas
- 1 avocado
- 4 eggs
- 2 tbsp whole milk
- ½ cup black beans
- ½ cup chunky salsa
- ½ tbsp butter

1. Place a skillet on a burner set to medium heat. Add the butter and wait for it to melt completely.
2. As the skillet heats up, crack four eggs into a bowl, add milk, and whisk vigorously.
3. Pour the egg mixture into the pan once the butter has completely melted.
4. Stir the eggs until curds begin to form. Add salt and pepper. You can continue to cook the eggs to your desired level of firmness.
5. While the eggs cook, cut the avocado in half, remove the pit, and peel the skin. Slice into lengthwise strips.
6. Place a tortilla on a flat surface. Spoon half the eggs into the tortilla and top with a few slices of the avocado. Scoop roughly half of the black beans and half of the salsa on top of the avocado.
7. Repeat for the second burrito.
8. To wrap, fold the far left and right edges of the burrito inwards. Then, roll the burrito towards you, laying the forward edge on top of the right and left edges. Finally fold the edge closest to you on top and roll the whole burrito away from your body.
9. Add the burrito, seam side down, to the hot pan to seal it shut and add a nice crunch to the tortilla.
10. Serve immediately and enjoy!

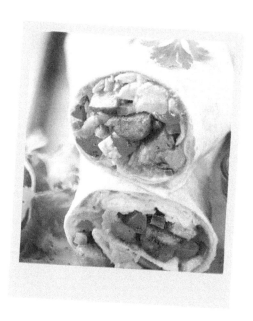

Fertility Omelet

Omelets are fantastic breakfast options for soon-to-be parents who want to start their day with ample protein and superfoods. You can make your omelet with any variation of your favorite ingredients, but the recipe below incorporates protein rich red meat, vitamin rich spinach, and full fat cheddar cheese to promote fertility.

The recipe below assumes the steak has already been cooked, so this recipe works well if you have leftovers from the night before. If you need to cook your steak at the moment, then season generously with salt and pepper before cooking for three to five minutes on each side in a hot skillet. Baste with butter and rosemary for an added burst of flavor.

Time: 17 minutes
Serving Size: 2
Prep Time: 5 minutes
Cook Time: 12 minutes
Nutritional Facts/Info:
554 calories, 30 g fat, 65 g protein, 2 g carbohydrates, 1 g sugar,

Ingredients:

- 4 eggs
- ½ cup chopped steak
- 1 cup spinach
- ½ cup cheddar cheese
- 1 tbsp butter
- Salt and pepper

1. Set a pan on the stove to medium heat. Add the butter and allow it to melt.
2. While the butter melts, crack four eggs into a small bowl and whisk vigorously. Season the eggs with salt and pepper to your taste.
3. Once the butter has fully melted, pour the egg mixture into the pan. Do not stir, instead, allow the bottom to cook fully. Pull the sides of the egg into the middle and tip the pan so the uncooked egg can reach the heat. Continue this process until very little uncooked egg remains on the top of the omelet.
4. Add the cooked steak, spinach and cheese to half of the omelet.
5. Fold the eggs in half and continue to cook for two to three minutes.
6. Carefully flip the omelet and continue to cook the other side for an additional two to three minutes.
7. Serve hot!

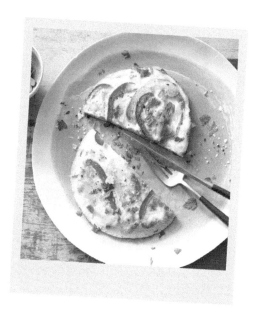

Yogurt Parfait

This is a great breakfast option for busy couples who want to incorporate fertility boosting foods into their daily routine without spending an hour in the kitchen in the morning. It is easy to double for two breakfasts. Using whole-fat yogurt is essential, as the nutrients from whole-fat dairy are key to boosting fertility.

Time: 5 minutes

Serving Size: 1

Prep Time: 5 minutes

Cook Time: 0 minutes

Nutritional Facts/Info:

264 calories, 13 g fat, 12 g protein, 28 g carbohydrates, 18 g sugar

Ingredients:

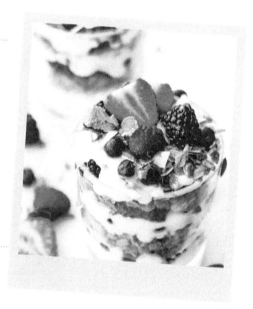

- 1 cup whole-fat yogurt
- ¼ cup blueberries
- ¼ raspberries
- 2 tbsp sunflower seeds
- ¼ cup plain or honey granola

Directions:

1. Scoop one cup of whole-fat yogurt into a bowl.
2. Thoroughly rinse the blueberries and raspberries before adding to the yogurt.
3. Sprinkle sunflower seeds and granola over top.
4. Enjoy!

Savory Oatmeal

Who says oatmeal has to be a sweet treat? If you aren't into sweet flavors like maple syrup or cinnamon at breakfast, that doesn't mean you have to give up the health benefits of oatmeal. Savory oatmeal is a great option to take advantage of the high fiber content and protein that can be built into a bowl of oatmeal. If you love spicy food, then you can increase the small portion of hot sauce included in this recipe. If spice isn't your thing, then feel free to exclude that ingredient.

Time: 12 minutes
Serving Size: 1
Prep Time: 2 minutes
Cook Time: 10 minutes
Nutritional Facts/Info:
685 calories, 38 g fat, 29 g protein, 62 g carbohydrates, 3 g sugar

Ingredients:

- ½ cup steel cut oats
- 1 egg
- ¼ cup great northern beans
- ¼ cup walnuts
- 2 tbsp hot sauce
- 1 tbsp butter
- 1 tsp cumin
- 1 tsp paprika
- Salt and pepper

1. Add steel cut oats and water to a bowl and microwave per package instructions.
2. Place a small frying pan on the stove and add butter. Allow it to melt.
3. Once the butter has melted, crack one egg into the pan. Season it with salt and pepper. Flip the egg after three to five minutes. Cook on the opposite side for two to three minutes.
4. Remove the fully cooked oatmeal from the microwave. Stir in great northern beans, hot sauce, cumin, paprika, and walnuts.
5. Top the oatmeal with the over-easy egg and enjoy!

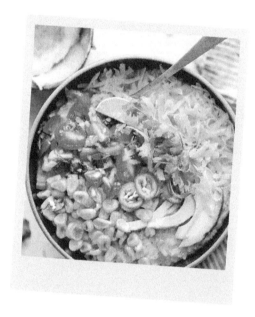

Fertility Friendly Pancakes

These health-conscious pancakes focus on bananas, rich in potassium, and oats, a complex carb, to increase fertility in both men and women. They are fall flavored and best served with your favorite maple syrup.

Time: 20 minutes

Serving Size: 2

Prep Time: 10 minutes

Cook Time: 10 minutes

Nutritional Facts/Info:

533 calories, 17 g fat, 11 g protein, 95 g carbohydrates, 23 g sugar

Ingredients:

- 3 bananas
- 1 ½ cups rolled oats
- 3 tsp baking powder
- 3 tbsp cinnamon
- 1 tsp ginger
- 1 tsp nutmeg
- 2 tbsp butter

Directions:

1. Peel the bananas and add them to a bowl. Mash the bananas until no lumps remain.
2. Add the dry ingredients to the mashed bananas and mix thoroughly.
3. Place a pan on the stovetop and set to medium heat. Add butter to the pan.
4. Once the butter has fully melted, scoop ¼ cups of the batter onto the pan and create a pancake sized disc.

5. Cook for three to five minutes on the first side before flipping and cooking on the opposite side for five minutes.

6. Remove from heat once fully cooked and serve warm with your favorite fertility friendly toppings.

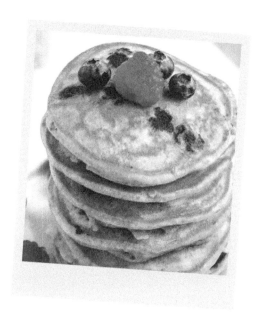

Banana Oat Muffins

These health-conscious and fertility friendly muffins rely on plant based proteins and full fat dairy options. They are easy to make ahead for grab-and-go breakfasts during the work week. Or, they are easy to throw together on a weekend with your partner.

Time: 50 minutes
Serving Size: 4
Prep Time: 15 minutes
Cook Time: 35 minutes
Nutritional Facts/Info:
410 calories, 5 g fat, 10 g protein, 87 g carbohydrates, 27 g sugar

Ingredients:

- 4 bananas
- 3 cups rolled oats
- 2 tbsp cinnamon
- 3 tsp baking powder
- ¼ cup whole-fat yogurt
- ¼ cup maple syrup or honey
- 1 tsp salt

Directions:

1. Preheat the oven to 350°F and line a muffin tin with paper cups.
2. Peel the bananas and add them to a bowl. Mash the bananas until no lumps remain.
3. Add the oats, cinnamon, baking powder, yogurt, syrup, and salt to the bowl. Mix until thoroughly incorporated.

4. Pour the mixture into the muffin tin, try and pour even amounts of batter into each cup.
5. Bake on the middle rack for 35 minutes.
6. Remove from the oven once fully cooked and allow to cool for five to ten minutes.
7. Enjoy warm!

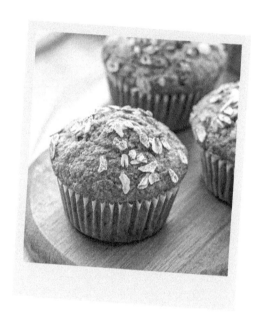

Protein Egg Bake

Egg bakes are like easy-to-cook quiches. You can pack them full of your favorite ingredients, in the case of this recipe that includes fertility friendly meats and dairies. If you prefer to meal prep your breakfasts, then this recipe is perfect for you! And, if you and your partner prefer different ingredients, that is fine too! Use some tinfoil to split your casserole dish in half, then place an egg mixture with your favorite ingredients on one side and a mixture with their favorite ingredients on the other side.

Time: 50 minutes

Serving Size: 6

Prep Time: 20 minutes

Cook Time: 30 minutes

Nutritional Facts/Info:

312 calories, 20 g fat, 32 g protein, 3 g carbohydrates, 2 g sugar

Ingredients:

- 9 eggs
- 1 cup onion
- 1 lb ground turkey
- ½ cup cheddar cheese
- ¼ cup whole milk
- 1 tbsp butter
- 1 tsp salt
- 1 tsp pepper
- ½ tsp garlic powder

Directions:

1. Preheat the oven to 350 °F.
2. In a bowl, crack and whisk the eggs. Add the milk once eggs are whisked and mix them together.
3. Place a pan on the stove top and add the butter. Once the butter has melted, place the ground turkey in the pan. Cook until the meat is completely cooked.
4. As the meat cooks, chop 1 onion and measure out 1 cup.
5. Remove the cooked meat from the stove and let it cool to room temperature.
6. Add the whisked eggs, onion, cheese, and meat to a casserole dish. Season the mixture with salt, pepper, and garlic powder. Stir until the ingredients and seasonings are evenly laid out.
7. Cook for 20 minutes or until the eggs are fluffy.
8. Enjoy warm and save for great breakfasts throughout the week!

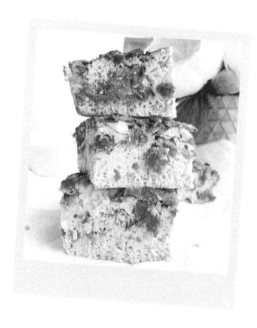

Southwest Scramble

An egg scramble is an easy way to feed two people breakfast. And this scramble includes kale, rich in folic acid, and red bell pepper, rich in vitamin E, both incredible foods for fertility. Not to mention the avocado! If you prefer spicy food, then increase the amount of chili powder you sprinkle onto the eggs while they cook. Or, add a few spoons of salsa to the finished product.

Time: 20 minutes
Serving Size: 2
Prep Time: 10 minutes
Cook Time: 10 minutes
Nutritional Facts/Info:
625 calories, 51 g fat, 32 g protein, 19 g carbohydrates, 3 g sugar

Ingredients:

- 6 eggs
- 1 cup kale
- ½ cup shredded mexican cheese mix
- ½ cup chopped red bell pepper
- 1 avocado
- 1 tsp salt
- 1 tsp pepper
- ½ tsp chili powder

Directions:

1. Wash and dry your vegetables prior to chopping.
2. Chop the kale into strips and chop the red bell pepper into one-inch cubes. You will likely not use the whole pepper. Save it for a later meal!
3. Cut the avocado in half, peel away the skin, and remove the pit. Cut the avocado into strips.
4. Place a pan on the stove top and add butter or oil.
5. While the pan heats, crack the six eggs into a bowl and whisk vigorously.
6. Once the butter has melted, add the kale and red bell pepper to the pan. Cook until the kale wilts, about five minutes, then turn the heat down to 'low' and pour the whisked eggs into the pan.
7. Stir constantly until the eggs are nearly cooked.
8. Top the scramble with cheese, salt, pepper, and chili powder. Continue to cook.
9. Remove from the pan once fully cooked. Place the scramble on your breakfast plate and top with the avocado slices. Enjoy with your morning coffee or OJ!

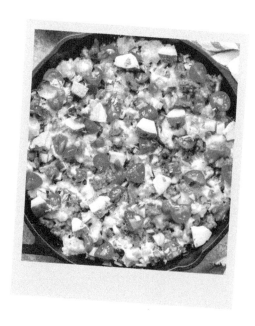

Fertility Fruit Salad

Fruit salad is a refreshing way to start the morning, though best served alongside a protein-filled dish for a well-rounded meal. The fruits included in this fruit salad all have a low glycemic-index. They are rich in the vitamins necessary to boost fertility in both men and women.

Time: 10 minutes

Serving Size: 5

Prep Time: 10 minutes

Cook Time: 10 minutes

Nutritional Facts/Info: 50 calories, 0 g fat, 1 g protein, 13 g carbohydrates, 10 g sugar

Ingredients:

- ½ cup blueberries
- ½ cup raspberries
- 1 cup watermelon
- ¼ cup pomegranates
- 1 cup plums

Directions:

1. Thoroughly wash all fruits before chopping.
2. Using a paring knife and a sturdy cutting board, cut the watermelon into 1 inch cubes. This can be easiest if starting from a pre-cut half or ¼ of a watermelon. Add watermelon cubes to a large bow.
3. Wipe extra liquid off the cutting board.
4. Cut and peel the plums into similarly sized one-inch cubes. Add these cubes to the bow.

5. Measure out and pour the blueberries, raspberries, and pomegranate seeds into the bowl.
6. Stir the fruits together until the bowl is well variegated.
7. Enjoy!

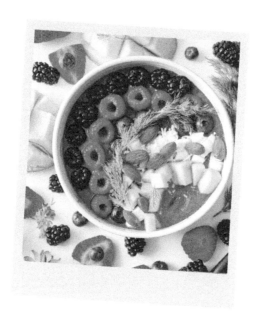

Blueberry Muffins

Muffins are a delicious treat in the morning, so a muffin with fertility benefits is even better. These muffins rely on gluten-free flour to reduce the amount of carbohydrates, and they include fertility superfoods like cinnamon. Muffins are a fun meal to prepare with your spouse on a lazy, weekend morning. They are also a good make ahead breakfast for the week.

Time: 30 minutes
Serving Size: 12
Prep Time: 10 minutes
Cook Time: 20 minutes
Nutritional Facts/Info: 152 calories, 2 g fat, 5 g protein, 30 g carbohydrates, 7 g sugar

Ingredients:

- 3 cups gluten-free flour
- 1 cup blueberries
- 3 eggs
- ¼ cup honey
- ½ tsp vanilla
- ½ tsp baking soda
- 1 tbsp cinnamon
- 1 tsp ginger
- ¼ tsp salt

1. Preheat the oven to 350 °F.
2. In a bowl, mix together flour, baking soda, cinnamon, ginger, and salt.
3. In a separate bowl, mix together eggs, honey, and vanilla.
4. Slowly dump the dry ingredients into the wet ingredients while stirring constantly. Once fully combined, add blueberries to the mixture.
5. Evenly scoop the mixture into muffin tins. For best results, only fill the muffin tins ½ to ¾ of the way. Overly filled muffin tins may take longer to bake.
6. Bake for 20 minutes.
7. Enjoy!

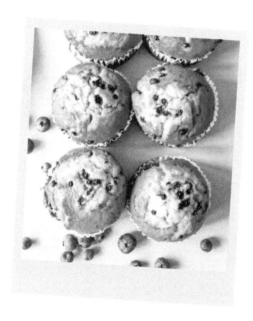

Citrus Sticky Rolls

Citrus fruits are an underrated fertility booster, and they are an easy inclusion into sticky rolls. Making sticky rolls can be a long-term morning (and overnight) project with your spouse, a great way to unwind, and a sweet treat to serve when friends or family are visiting. If you are looking for fertility recipes around the holidays, then these are perfect for a fertility filled Christmas morning.

Time: 8 hours and 20 minutes

Serving Size: 8

Prep Time: 8 hours

Cook Time: 20 minutes

Nutritional Facts/Info:

447 calories, 27 g fat, 7 g protein, 40 g carbohydrates, 42 g sugar

Dough Ingredients:

- 1 cup whole milk
- 2 tsp active dry yeast
- ¼ cup honey
- ¼ cup brown sugar
- 2 eggs
- 4 cups almond flour
- 1 ½ tsp salt
- 6 tbsp butter
- **Filling Ingredients:**
- ½ cup butter
- 2 tbsp cinnamon
- ¼ cup orange zest
- ½ cup brown sugar

Frosting Ingredients:

- 4 ounces cream cheese
- 4 tbsp butter
- 4 tbsp orange juice
- 1 tsp lemon juice
- 1 1/2 cups powdered sugar

Directions:

1. Begin by creating the dough. Warm the milk in a microwave for 20 to 30 seconds, then pour it into the bowl of a stand mixer. Add the sugar and yeast. Allow those ingredients to stand for five minutes.
2. Place the stand mixer on a low setting. Add the eggs, honey, flour, and salt to the mixture.
3. Once those ingredients are well incorporated, slowly add the butter to the bowl. This works best if the butter is extremely soft, but not melted.
4. Leave the mixer kneading on medium speed for six more minutes.
5. Wipe a separate bowl with oil and transfer the dough to the oiled bowl. Cover with plastic wrap and place in the refrigerator for five to eight hours.
6. In the morning, remove the dough from the fridge. Place it on a clean, floured surface and roll out until it is ½ inch thick.
7. In a bowl, combine the filling ingredients butter, cinnamon, orange zest, and brown sugar. They should form a sandy mixture.
8. Spread the mixture across the rolled out dough so that it is even.
9. Once spread, begin to roll the dough, working slowly. It will eventually form a long rope-like shape with a spiral visible on either end. If the spiral isn't visible, you can chop off the misshapen ends.
10. Next, you need to cut the dough into eight equal discs. You can use a knife or scissors, but for best results use dental floss or string. The floss or string will maintain the spiral and shape of the roll best. Take the floss or string and slide it under the roll. Find the middle of the roll, hold the string up so it is equal lengths in each hand,

cross it over and pull until it has broken all the way through the roll. Repeat this process, cutting the rolls in half until you have eight cinnamon rolls.

11. Arrange the eight rolls in a 9 x 13 baking dish, cover with a dish towel, and allow them to rise for an additional hour.

12. Once risen, preheat the oven to 350 °F and bake for 20 minutes. If you like your rolls on the gooey side, then pull them from the oven around 18 minutes.

13. Make the frosting while the rolls bake. In the bowl of a stand mixer, combine the cream cheese, butter, orange juice, and lemon juice. Mix well.

14. Slowly add the sugar while the stand mixer is on a low setting.

15. Remove the rolls from the oven and allow to cool for five to ten minutes.

16. Once cooled, generously top with the citrus frosting.

17. Serve warm and enjoy!

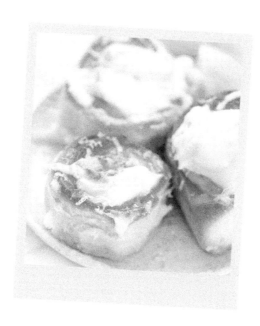

Quiche

Eating quiche is like eating pie for breakfast! In this case, the pie is packed with protein that soon-t0-be parents need in order to boost their fertility. You are more than welcome to get experimental in the kitchen and make your own pie crust, but a store bought variety will do perfectly for this recipe too. Be sure not to skip step five, pre-baking the crust in the oven, otherwise it may be difficult to achieve a crisp pie crust all the way around.

Time: 45 minutes

Serving Size: 6

Prep Time: 10 minutes

Cook Time: 35 minutes

Nutritional Facts/Info:

319 calories, 17 g fat, 27 g protein, 13 g carbohydrates, 3 g sugar

Ingredients:

- 1 frozen pie crust
- 6 eggs
- ½ cup milk
- ½ onion
- 1 cup chopped steak
- ½ cup cheddar cheese
- 2 tsp salt
- 1 tsp pepper
- 1 tsp garlic powder
- 1 scoop collagen peptide powder

1. Preheat the oven to 350 °F.
2. Using a cutting board and a sharp knife, chop half of one white onion. Then, slice a steak into one-inch cubes.
3. In a bowl, whisk six eggs and milk together. Season the mixture with salt, pepper, and garlic powder. Add the collagen peptide powder.
4. Add the onion, steak, and cheese to the egg mixture.
5. Add the empty pie crust to the oven and bake for five minutes. Then, remove it from the oven.
6. Pour the egg mixture into the pie crust.
7. Bake for 30 minutes or per pie crust package instructions.
8. When the quiche is finished baking, the eggs should have a pillowy consistency, fully cooked boot moveable.
9. Cut into slices and enjoy!

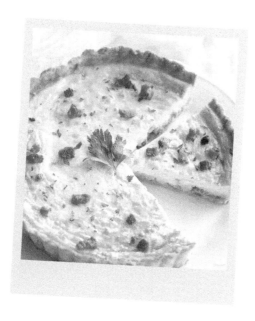

Breakfast Meat Scramble

This recipe is a great solution for carnivores who don't want to skip the meat at breakfast. It includes liver, the fertility superfood, and spinach which is rich in the vitamins and nutrients that men and women need when conceiving. Since everything is cooked in the same pan, you'll be saving time on dishes that you can spend on more important things. This recipe is best cooked in a cast iron skillet, but a standard frying pan will work as well.

Time: 35 minutes
Serving Size: 4
Prep Time: 10 minutes
Cook Time: 25 minutes
Nutritional Facts/Info:
610 calories, 36 g fat, 47 g protein, 24 g carbohydrates, 2 g sugar

Ingredients:

- ½ cup beef liver
- 4 strips bacon
- 4 sausage links
- 8 eggs
- 1 cup spinach
- ½ cup cheddar cheese
- 4 slices sourdough bread
- 2 tbsp butter
- Salt and pepper

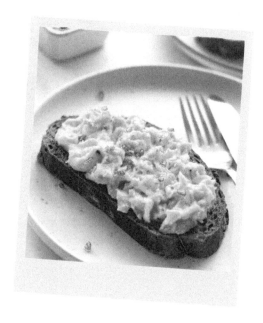

Directions:

1. In a skillet on the stove, place the butter to melt. Once melted add the bacon to the pan. Cook the bacon until stiff, flipping as you go, it should take roughly ten minutes.
2. Chop the sausage links into one-inch chunks.
3. Remove the cooked bacon from the pan and replace with the sausage and liver.
4. Cook the sausage and liver for roughly ten minutes, stirring as you go, or until cooked thoroughly.
5. While the meats cook, chop the bacon into bite sized pieces. Crack the eggs into a bowl and whisk until smooth. Season the eggs with salt and pepper.
6. Toast the slices of bread into the toaster or under the oven broiler and toast to your preference.
7. Place the bacon back in the pan and add the spinach. Stir the meat and greens until the spinach begins to wilt.
8. Move the meat and greens to one side of the pan and turn down the heat to low. Pour the eggs into the open side of the pan. Gently stir the eggs until they form curds and scramble. Do not allow them to mix with the meats and greens. Top the eggs with the cheese. Continue to cook the eggs to your preference.
9. Arrange the cooked meat and greens, eggs, and toast on your breakfast plate. Enjoy by combining the foods, adding meat and eggs to the bread, or separately.

Breakfast Sandwich

Breakfast sandwiches are delicious and customizable breakfast options that we've managed to twist into a fertility powerhouse. You can make adjustments to this recipe as needed, like swapping out the Everything Bagel for your favorite breakfast bread or using your favorite cheese. But, don't skip that iron rich red-meat or the fertility friendly avocado!

Time: 20 minutes
Serving Size: 1
Prep Time: 5 minutes
Cook Time: 15 minutes
Nutritional Facts/Info:
744 calories, 35 g fat, 75 g protein, 32 g carbohydrates, 5 g sugar

Ingredients:

- 1 everything bagel
- 2 eggs
- 2 slices of your favorite cheese
- 1 small steak filet
- ½ avocado
- 1 scoop collagen peptide powder
- 2 tbsp butter
- Salt and pepper

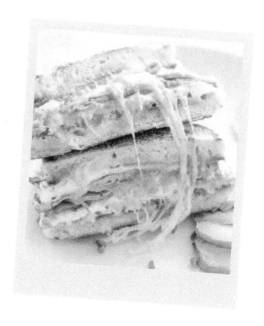

1. Place the halves of the bagel into a toaster or under the oven broiler to toast.
2. Season the steak filet with salt and pepper.
3. In a pan on a high burner, add the butter and allow it to melt. Once melted, place the steak on the pan.
4. Cook the meat for 3 minutes on each side.
5. Once cooked fully, remove the steak from the pan. While the pan is still on the stove, crack both eggs into it and allow them to cook on one side for three to five.
6. As the eggs cook, slice the steak filet into smaller pieces. You will have leftover steak.
7. Flip the eggs and cook on the opposite side for two to three minutes.
8. Cut an avocado in half, remove the pit and skin. Place half the avocado in a bowl with a scoop of collagen peptide powder and mash the two together until fully incorporated.
9. Remove the bagel from the toaster or broiler, arrange on a plate and top with the fried eggs, cheese slices, steak slices, and avocado mixture.
10. Enjoy!

Breakfast Bars

These homemade granola bars are a perfect grab-and-go breakfast. They're sweet and packed with the vitamins and nutrients that soon-to-be parents need in their diet. Make this as a side for your Saturday morning breakfast feast, or make them ahead and save for quick breakfasts all week. The health benefits in these bars can be enjoyed by him and her!

Time: 35 minutes

Serving Size: 12

Prep Time: 5 minutes

Cook Time: 30 minutes

Nutritional Facts/Info: 133 calories, 6 g fat, 4 g protein, 19 g carbohydrates, 6 g sugar

Ingredients:

- 2 cups rolled oats
- 1 banana
- ½ cup whole milk
- 2 tbsp cinnamon
- ½ cup walnuts
- ½ cup dark chocolate chips
- ½ cup pomegranate seeds

Directions:

1. Preheat the oven to 400 °F.
2. In a bowl, mash the banana. Add the oats, milk, and cinnamon. Stir together until combined.

3. Add the walnuts, pomegranates, and chocolate chips to the mixture. Stir together until the ingredients are evenly distributed.
4. Pour the mixture into a 9 x 13 casserole dish and bake in the oven for 30 minutes.
5. Remove from the oven and allow to cool before cutting into 12 even squares.
6. Enjoy immediately or store in the fridge for up to five days!

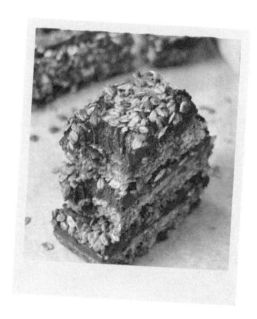

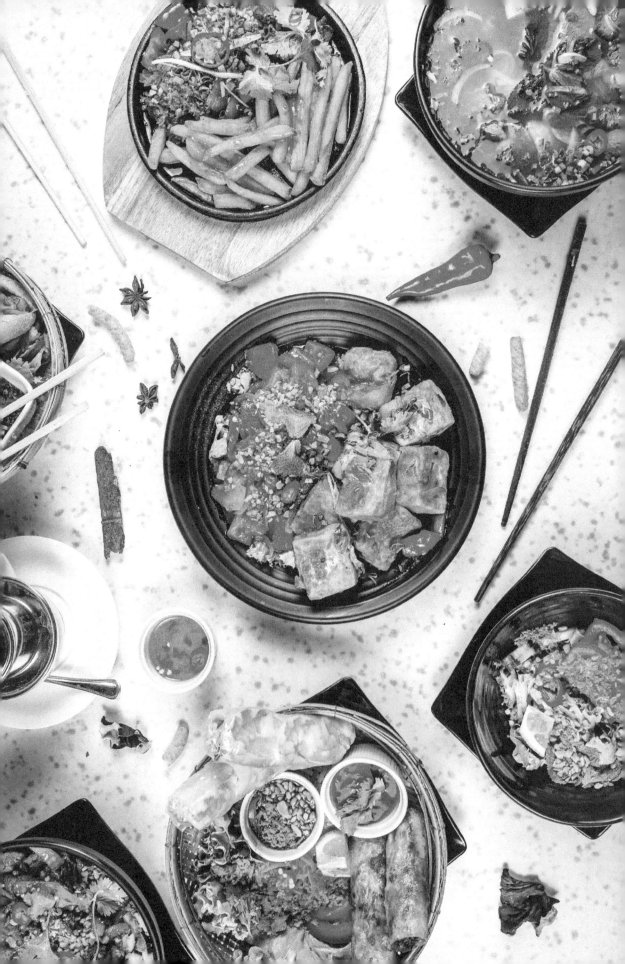

CHAPTER FOUR

Lunch

———

Lunch can be hard to cook for, and many people end up with nothing but leftovers and snacks. However, there are dozens of great, quick, and simple recipes that are packed with fertility friendly ingredients and make for a tasty lunch. The increasing popularity of working from home has revolutionized the way you can eat lunch. Don't rule out one of the recipes below just because it takes more than 30 minutes to cook! Sometimes taking a lesson from the French and slowing down for lunch is a great opportunity to connect with family and eat good food. Taste test a few of my favorites like the steak curry, salmon and rice bowl, or southwest salad! The recipes below rely heavily on spinach, chickpeas, and avocados. The nutrients found in these foods like protein, Vitamin A, and focate are key for reproductive health. These recipes will continue to benefit a growing fetus too, remember that everything the mother eats during pregnancy is passed right on to the fetus. Keep up the healthy fertility diet through all nine months of your pregnancy and conception journey for best results.

For best results, you'll want to make sure you have all the right tools in the kitchen. The most common tools required in these recipes are a microwave, pots and pans, cutting board, a sharp knife for cutting vegetables, and small bowls or measuring cups for making salad dressing.

Fertility Protein Bowl

This protein bowl is simple to throw together for lunch during a workday, especially if you keep the sweet potato and quinoa cooked ahead of time. It combines the fertility boosting power of lentils with so many other healthy vegetables. Make ahead of time if you like to meal prep or share with your partner on the weekends.

Serving Size: 2
Prep Time: 25 minutes
Cook Time: Varies
Nutritional Facts/Info:
873 calories, 57 g fat, 19 g protein, 79 g carbohydrates, 17 g sugar

Bowl Ingredients:

- ¼ cup diced carrot
- ¼ cup yellow bell pepper
- ¼ cup cucumber
- ¼ cup chickpeas
- ¼ black beans
- ¼ cherry tomatoes
- ¼ cup baked sweet potato
- ½ cup quinoa
- ½ cup shredded red cabbage

Dressing Ingredients:

- ½ cup olive oil
- ¼ cup balsamic vinegar
- 1 tbsp dijon mustard

- 1 tbsp honey
- Salt and pepper

Directions:

1. If you don't have baked sweet potatoes prepared ahead of time, then begin this recipe by preheating the oven, adding chopped sweet potato to a baking sheet, and baking for 25 to 30 minutes.
2. Chop the bell pepper, cucumber, tomatoes, and carrots into one-inch or smaller cubes.
3. If you don't have pre-cooked quinoa prepared ahead of time, then add your quinoa to a pot on the stove and cook to package instructions.
4. To prepare the dressing, add olive oil, balsamic vinegar, mustard, and honey to a mason jar. Screw on the lid and shake vigorously for one to two minutes.
5. To assemble the protein bowl, add the carrot, bell pepper, cucumber, chickpeas, black beans, tomato, quinoa, sweet potato, and shredded cabbage to a bowl. Drizzle with the dressing and enjoy!

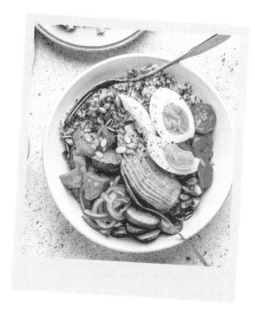

Salmon and Rice Bowl

The only (and best) use of leftover salmon, or fresh if you have a long lunch planned, that you'll ever need. This dish makes it possible to have fertility boosting salmon, even at lunch. It is easy to meal prep and you can easily double this recipe when making lunch for two.

Serving Size: 1
Prep Time: 3 minutes
Cook Time: Varies
Nutritional Facts/Info:
964 calories, 35 g fat, 76 g protein, 86 g carbohydrates, 1 g sugar

Ingredients:

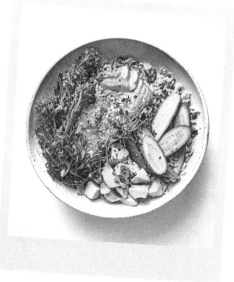

- ½ cup sliced salmon
- ¼ cup rice or quinoa
- ½ avocado
- 2 tbsp sriracha
- 2 tbsp soy sauce

Directions:

1. If using pre-cooked salmon and rice, put both in a bowl and microwave for 90 seconds.
2. Once heated, add sliced avocado and drizzle with sriracha and soy sauce.
3. If you need to cook the salmon and rice for this dish, then bake the salmon for 10 to 12 minutes. Cook the rice in a pot on the stove burner per package directions. Then top with the other ingredients as before.

Steak Sandwich

These filling sandwiches can be made on the grill for a fun Saturday afternoon cookout, or inside on the stove top. They are filling, packed with protein and nutrients, and will boost fertility for both him and her. Onions in particular are great for enhancing men's sperm quality. Don't skimp there!

Time: 20 minutes

Serving Size: 2

Prep Time: 10 minutes

Cook Time: 10 minutes

Nutritional Facts/Info:

1,728 calories, 78 g fat, 199 g protein, 51 g carbohydrates, 5 g sugar

Ingredients:

- 1 lb strip steak
- 1 cup shredded mozzarella cheese
- 1 cup kale
- ½ onion
- 2 hoagie rolls
- Salt and pepper

Directions:

1. Preheat a grill or skillet to medium high heat, add butter to grease if necessary.
2. Slice the onion into long, thin strips.
3. Season the strip steak slices with salt and pepper.
4. Add the onion to the hot skillet and cook until translucent.
5. Move the onion to the side to continue cooking and add the slices of steak to the skillet or grill.

6. Cook the steak slices for two minutes on one side before tossing and cooking for an additional three minutes on the other side.

7. While the meat and veggies cook, cut the hoagie rolls in half. Place them under the broiler for two to three minutes.

8. Remove the steak and onions from the skillet.

9. Remove the hoagie rolls from the broiler.

10. To assemble the sandwich, place mozzarella directly on the toasted bun and quickly top with the still hot meat and onions. This will naturally melt the cheese. Top with a handful of kale and the top of the hoagie roll.

11. These can be enjoyed on their own or served with one of the delicious snacks from Chapter 8.

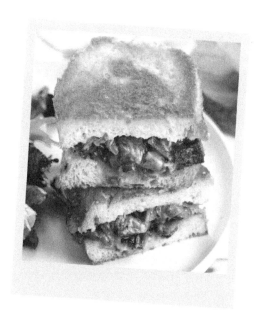

Quinoa and Sweet Potato Bowl

These easy lunch bowls serve two, and they are perfect for a weekend lunch around the house. They can easily be meal prepped if they become a favorite you want to enjoy again and again. The dark leafy green kale is full of fertility friendly vitamins. The addition of quinoa, a healthy carb, and chickpeas as a plant-based protein source, round out these delicious lunches.

Time: 45 minutes

Serving Size: 2

Prep Time: 15 minutes

Cook Time: 30 minutes

Nutritional Facts/Info:

840 calories, 34 g fat, 31 g protein, 108 g carbohydrates, 11 g sugar

Ingredients:

- 1 sweet potato
- ½ cup chickpeas
- 1 cup quinoa
- ¼ cup shredded red cabbage
- cup feta cheese
- ¼ cup almonds
- 2 cups kale
- 2 tbsp lemon juice
- 2 tbsp olive oil
- Salt and pepper

Directions:

1. Preheat the oven to 375 °F.
2. Chop the sweet potato into one-inch cubes and arrange them on a baking sheet.
3. Coat in olive oil, salt, and pepper, then bake for 30 minutes.
4. While the sweet potato bakes, place a pot of water on the stove and turn to medium heat.
5. Cook the quinoa per package directions.
6. Allow the sweet potatoes and quinoa to cool once fully cooked.
7. To assemble the salad, lay the kale in the bottom of the bowls. Top with quinoa, chopped sweet potatoes, chickpeas, red cabbage, feta, and almonds. Drizzle in lemon juice, olive oil, salt, and pepper. Enjoy!

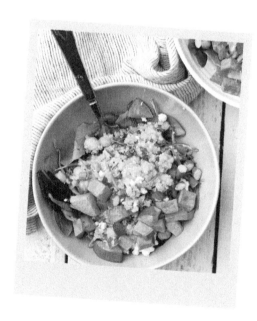

Super Salad

Salads are delicious and nutritious ways to pack in lots of fertility boosting ingredients. This salad starts with a dark, leafy green base and includes five fertility friendly foods. It can be assembled in less than 15 minutes, making it a perfect and quick lunch. It can also be added to a mason jar for lunch meal prepping.

Time: 15 minutes

Serving Size: 1

Prep Time: 5 minutes

Cook Time: 10 minutes

Nutritional Facts/Info:

513 calories, 15 g fat, 32 g protein, 66 g carbohydrates, 14 g sugar

Dry Ingredients:

- 1 cup spinach
- 2 eggs
- ½ cup chickpeas
- ½ cup cherry tomatoes

Dressing Ingredients:

- 3 tbsp olive oil
- 2 tbsp dijon mustard
- 1 clove garlic
- 2 tbsp white wine vinegar
- Salt and pepper

1. Place a pot to boil on the stove. Once the water is boiling, add the two eggs. Immediately cut the heat, but leave the eggs in the water for eight minutes.
2. Remove the eggs from the water and rinse in cold water. Remove the shells and chop them into bite sized pieces.
3. In a small bowl, combine the dressing ingredients and whisk until smooth.
4. In a larger bowl, place the spinach leaves, chickpeas, eggs, and tomatoes. Top with dressing and enjoy!

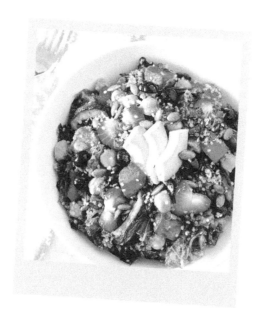

Veggie Wrap

When following a fertility diet, wraps can be a great substitution for sandwiches. Some gluten-based carbs are fine, but if you are splurging on muffins or pancakes in the morning, you may want to avoid heavy breads for the rest of the day. This wrap is low-carb, and is stuffed with fertility friendly ingredients that will keep you full throughout the day. Even better? There's no cooking involved!

Time: 10 minutes
Serving Size: 1
Prep Time: 10 minutes
Cook Time: 0 minutes
Nutritional Facts/Info:
1,109 calories, 63 g fat, 30 g protein, 106 g carbohydrates, 17 g sugar

Ingredients:

- 1 spinach wrap
- ½ cup chickpeas
- ½ cup spinach
- ¼ cup chopped tomatoes
- ¼ cup chopped cucumber
- ¼ cup green goddess dressing

Directions:

1. Open a can of chickpeas, drain them into a strainer and rinse with cold water. Pat the chickpeas dry with a paper towel and set aside.
2. Chop one tomato into one-inch cubes until you have roughly ¼ cup. There will be leftover tomatoes. Do the same with a cucumber, there will be leftover cucumber too.

3. Place the spinach wrap flat spread green goddess dressing over it. Top with spinach, chickpeas, tomatoes, and cucumber. Drizzle with the remaining green goddess dressing.

4. To fold, hold the edges of the spinach wrap closest to your body and press forward continually. Roll into a long, cylindrical tube.

5. Enjoy! And, save the leftover chickpeas, tomatoes, and cucumber for the next day's lunch!

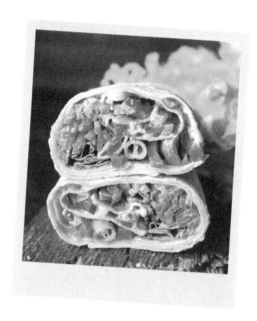

Chicken Liver Quesadilla

Quesadillas are delicious, cheesy, and warm. They make a great lunch on the weekends, or a great lunch for remote workers with easy access to their kitchen during the day. You can easily double or even triple this recipe if you are cooking for more than one person. It perfectly follows the fertility diet, giving dieters the vitamins and nutrients found in chicken liver and the full fat dairy of cheese.

Time: 35 minutes

Serving Size: 1

Prep Time: 5 minutes

Cook Time: 30 minutes

Nutritional Facts/Info:

347 calories, 13 g fat, 34 g protein, 24 g carbohydrates, 1 g sugar

Ingredients:

- 2 corn tortillas
- ½ cup shredded quesadilla cheese
- ¼ lb chicken liver
- 2 tbsp hot sauce
- 2 tbsp butter
- Salt and pepper

Directions:

1. If working with uncooked chicken liver, season with salt and pepper before placing in a pan to cook for five minutes on one side. Flip and continue cooking for seven minutes on the opposite side. You can also cook your chicken liver in the oven at 350 °F for 25 minutes, or poached for 15 minutes.

2. Once the chicken liver is cooked, remove from heat and shred with two forks. You will only need a bit of this filet of chicken liver. Set aside the rest for future lunches.
3. In a clean pan, melt the butter over a burner on medium heat.
4. Once melted, place one tortilla in the pan, add cheese, hot sauce, and the chicken liver. Sprinkle more cheese over top of the chicken liver so it is mostly covered, and then place the second tortilla on top.
5. Cook for four minutes and then flip to cook on the other side for four to six minutes.
6. Remove the quesadilla from the heat. Allow the quesadilla to cool for a few minutes and then cut into fourths.
7. Enjoy!

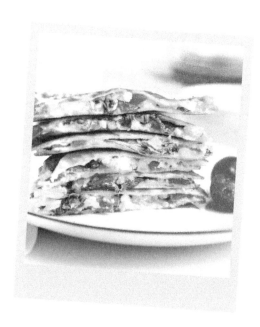

Southwest Salad

If you like your food on the spicy side, then dive into this tangy southwest salad. The fertility boosting ingredients of beans and spinach will provide the lean protein and vitamins that soon-to-be parents need to balance their hormones and strengthen their reproductive systems. You can choose your favorite pepper to add to this recipe, jalapenos will give it an extra kick and green peppers will add some sweetness.

Time: 15 minutes

Serving Size: 2

Prep Time: 15 minutes

Cook Time: 0 minutes

Nutritional Facts/Info:

688 calories, 21 g fat, 34 g protein, 96 g carbohydrates, 4 g sugar

Salad Ingredients:

- 3 cups mixed spinach and kale
- 1 cup black beans
- ½ cup shredded cheddar cheese
- ½ cup chopped tomatoes
- ¼ cup chopped peppers
- ¼ cup crushed tortilla chips

Dressing Ingredients:

- ¼ cup hot sauce
- ¼ cup mayonnaise
- 2 tbsp mustard
- 2 tbsp vinegar
- Salt and pepper

1. Begin by chopping the pepper and tomato into bite-sized chunks. You can remove the seeds from any pepper to lessen the spice. Reserve the remaining tomato and pepper for later lunches.

2. Place two or three tortilla chips in a plastic bag and crush with your hands or a rolling pin. Set aside.

3. In a bowl, combine the hot sauce, mayonnaise, mustard, vinegar, salt, and pepper. Stir until it is one homogenous mixture. If you would like a thinner dressing, add in a few tablespoons of water until you have reached the desired consistency.

4. To assemble the salad, place 1.5 cups of the greens into one bowl. You will repeat all of these steps for the second salad. Top with the beans, tomatoes, peppers, cheese, and crushed tortilla chips. Drizzle the dressing overtop.

5. Enjoy!

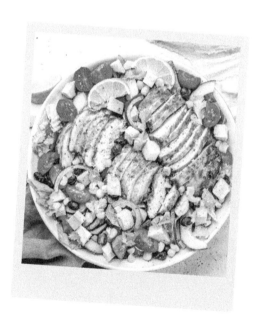

Salmon Pinwheels

This recipe works best when you have leftover tuna to quickly throw together during lunch, but it is possible to make your salmon during lunch too. These pinwheels are packed with fertility boosting ingredients. They are easy to make, and can feed a crowd as well as just one by reducing or doubling the recipe.

Time: 10 minutes

Serving Size: 2

Prep Time: 10 minutes

Cook Time: Varies

Nutritional Facts/Info: 269 calories, 6 g fat, 14 g protein, 39 g carbohydrates, 3 g sugar

Ingredients:

- ½ salmon filet
- ¼ cup whole-fat plain yogurt
- ¼ cup green onions
- 2 tbsp lemon juice
- 3 tortillas
- 1 tsp dill

Directions:

1. If you need to cook the salmon prior to assembling the pinwheels, then begin by preheating your oven to 350 °F. Drizzle the salmon filet with lemon juice and season with salt. Cook for 12 minutes.
2. If you are beginning with pre-cooked salmon, or once your salmon is cooked, separate the meat from the skin. Place the meat in a bowl and shred using two forks.
3. Chop the green onions into ½ inch pieces.

4. Mix the shredded salmon with yogurt, green onions, lemon juice, and dill. It should form a sticky paste that is mostly salmon.
5. Generously smear the tortillas with the mixture.
6. Roll the tortillas as you would a wrap, grabbing the tortilla side closest to you and folding forward until you have a cylinder.
7. Using a sharp knife, slice into the cylinder every two inches. Continue for each of the tortillas until you have a platter of pinwheels. They should resemble spirals once cut.
8. Enjoy immediately or save extras for future lunches.

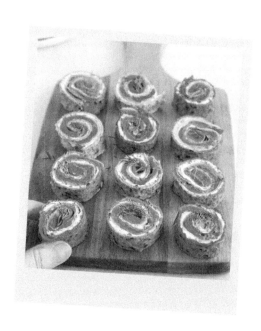

Egg Salad Sandwich

Eggs are one of the best foods for soon-to-be parents. They are rich in protein, vitamin B, and vitamin E. These sandwiches offer a unique way to get your day's serving of eggs. It is a great summer food option too!

Time: 22 minutes

Serving Size: 1

Prep Time: 10 minutes

Cook Time: 12 minutes

Nutritional Facts/Info:

665 calories, 47 g fat, 32 g protein, 36 g carbohydrates, 8 g sugar

Ingredients:

- 3 eggs
- 2 slices bread
- ¼ cup whole-fat plain yogurt
- ¼ cup mustard
- ½ avocado
- Salt and pepper

Directions:

1. Place a pot of water to boil on the stove.
2. Once boiling, add the whole eggs to the water and immediately cut the heat. Allow the eggs to sit in the water for eight minutes.
3. While the eggs cook, cut the avocado in half. Remove the skins and pit and then set aside.

4. Remove the hard boiled eggs from the water and immediately rinse in cold water. Peel away the egg shell and place the eggs onto a cutting board.

5. Chop the hard boiled eggs into one-inch cubes.

6. In a bowl, mash half of the avocado. Once smooth, add the yogurt and mustard to the bowl. Stir the ingredients until they are fully incorporated. Add salt and pepper.

7. Stir the egg cubes into the mixture until they are thoroughly coated.

8. Spoon the egg mixture onto the slices of bread and stack to create a sandwich.

9. Enjoy!

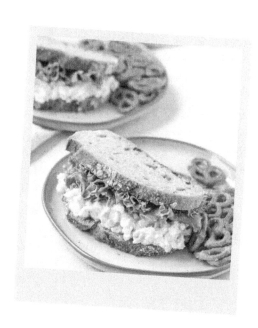

Bean Burger

This recipe not only follows the fertility diet, but it is also vegan. So, if you are attempting to follow a fertility diet and adhering to a dietary restriction, this is the lunch for you! The lean proteins from the beans and the vitamins and nutrients that come from the additional vegetables create an incredibly healthy lunch. Make these burgers on a Saturday afternoon or prepare them ahead of time for your meal-planned lunches.

Time: 40 minutes

Serving Size: 4

Prep Time: 20 minutes

Cook Time: 20 minutes

Nutritional Facts/Info: 271 calories, 3 g fat, 9 g protein, 52 g carbohydrates, 5 g sugar

Ingredients:

- 1 can black beans
- 1 yellow onion
- 1 tbsp minced garlic
- ½ cup grated carrots
- ¼ cup green bell pepper
- ¾ cup flour
- 1 tbsp cornstarch
- 1 tbsp water
- 2 tsp chili powder
- 2 tsp cumin
- 1 tsp salt
- 1 tsp pepper
- Burger buns and your favorite toppings

1. Preheat the oven to 350 °F.
2. Using a sharp knife and a cutting board, chop the garlic and green pepper into ¼ inch pieces. If the carrots are not yet grated, then grate ½ cup of carrots.
3. Drain the can of beans and add them to a bowl. Mash the beans until smooth.
4. Add the onion, carrots, peppers, and garlic to the bowl. Stir until the ingredients are evenly distributed.
5. In a separate bowl, stir together the cornstarch and water. Once combined add the chili powder, cumin, salt, and pepper to the mixture.
6. Add the cornstarch mixture to the bowl of vegetables .
7. Stir the flour into the mixture, slowly, so it incorporates slowly. The mixture should become a sticky batter.
8. Mold patty-sized discs out of the mixture and place them on a baking sheet.
9. Cook for 10 minutes, flip, and cook for another ten minutes.
10. Remove the patties from the oven and assemble the burgers with buns and your favorite toppings. For toppings that yield the best fertility results, top your burger with spinach, tomatoes, and avocado.
11. Enjoy!

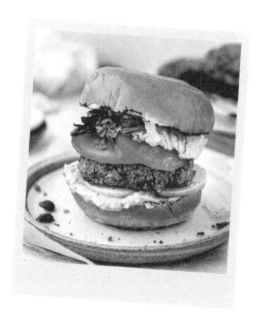

Greek Wrap

Make lunch for two! These fertility friendly wraps are filled with chickpeas, spinach, and lean proteins to help soon-to-be parents improve their fertility health and balance their hormones. Working from home? This lunch is easy and quick to assemble with your partner. Working in the office? It is easy to prep the ingredients ahead of time and bring this wrap with you, anywhere.

Time: 25 minutes
Serving Size: 2
Prep Time: 15 minutes
Cook Time: 10 minutes
Nutritional Facts/Info:
996 calories, 46 g fat, 53 g protein, 104 g carbohydrates, 29 g sugar

Ingredients:

- 1 can chickpeas
- cup tahini
- 3 tbsp water
- 2 tbsp olive oil
- 1 tsp cumin
- 1 tsp salt
- 1 tsp pepper
- 2 tbsp garlic
- 1 lemon
- 2 flour tortillas
- 1 cup spinach
- 2 tbsp honey
- ½ lb chicken breast

Directions:

1. Season the chicken breast with salt and pepper.
2. Place a pan on the stove to medium heat and add butter to the pan. Allow the butter to melt. Once it has melted, add the chicken breast to the pan. Cook the chicken for five minutes on one side.
3. While the chicken cooks, drain the can of chickpeas. Pour the chickpeas into a strainer and rinse in cool water. Set them aside.
4. In a food processor, add tahini, water, olive oil, cumin, salt, garlic, and lemon juice. Turn on the food processor to a medium speed and blend until smooth. About 20 seconds.
5. Add the chickpeas to the food processor and pulse to puree the entire mixture. Continue pulsing for three to four minutes. Scrape down the sides as needed to ensure all of the ingredients are thoroughly combined.
6. Adjust the seasonings as needed for your ideal taste.
7. Scoop the hummus out of the food processor and set aside.
8. Flip the chicken to cook the other side for five to seven minutes.
9. Remove the chicken from the heat and place in a bowl.
10. Once the chicken has cooled, use two forks to shred the chicken. You can make the shredded pieces as large or small as you'd like.
11. To assemble the wrap, place a tortilla flat on a plate. Smear the hummus across the tortilla, then top with the spinach and chicken. Drizzle honey overtop. Then, grabbing the side of the tortilla closest to you, fold forward until you have formed a cylindrical tube.
12. Repeat the assembly process for the second wrap.
13. Enjoy!

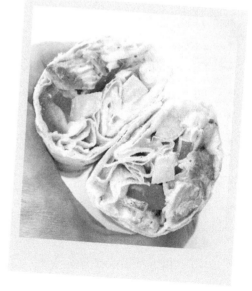

Chicken and Kale Salad

This fertility boosting salad is made up of nutritious greens and lean proteins to keep you powered up after the lunch hour. It is easy to assemble, especially if you are working with leftover chicken. We've included a dressing recipe below, but you can easily buy a tangy dressing from the grocery store that will complement this salad beautifully.

Time: 27 minutes

Serving Size: 1

Prep Time: 15 minutes

Cook Time: 12 minutes

Nutritional Facts/Info:

448 calories, 17 g fat, 50 g protein, 23 g carbohydrates, 3 g sugar

Salad Ingredients:

- 2 cups kale
- 2 chicken tenders
- ½ cup dried cranberries
- ¼ cup Parmesan
- 1 lemon
- 1 tsp salt

Dressing Ingredients:

- ¼ cup olive oil
- ¼ cup soy sauce
- 2 tbsp brown mustard
- 2 tbsp honey
- 1 tsp salt

- 1 tbsp lemon juice
- 1 tsp pepper

Directions:

1. Measure out 2 cups of kale, rinse the leaves, then add them to a salad bowl. Season the kale with salt and the juice of one lemon before massaging the leaves like you would a dough ball. This will enhance the flavor of the kale and make for a better meal.
2. If you are starting with leftover chicken, skip this step. Otherwise, season two raw chicken tenders with salt and pepper. Place a pan on the stove to medium heat and add olive oil to the pan. Once hot, add the chicken to the pan and sear on both sides, roughly five to seven minutes per side. Remove the chicken from the pan and slice into thin pieces.
3. In a small bowl, whisk together all of the dressing ingredients, using the remaining juice from the earlier lemon if possible. After whisking, the dressing should be light yellow and a syrupy consistency.
4. To assemble the salad, top the seasoned kale with the dried cranberries, sliced chicken, and Parmesan. Drizzle the dressing over the whole bowl.
5. Enjoy!

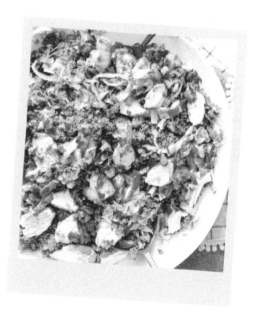

The Ultimate Fertility Diet Sandwich

This isn't just any sandwich, this sandwich is packed with four fertility boosting foods. This sandwich works best for lunch when using pre-cooked pork belly. See chapter 6 for a delicious pork belly dinner recipe, when you have leftovers from the night before you can assemble this sandwich in no time! You can use any bread for this sandwich, but we recommend something hearty, like a hoagie roll or other baguette.

Time: 10 minutes

Serving Size: 2

Prep Time: 5 minutes

Cook Time: 5 minutes

Nutritional Facts/Info:

1,405 calories, 105 g fat, 89 g protein, 28 g carbohydrates, 6 g sugar

Ingredients:

- 2 cups spinach
- 8 oz mozzarella cheese
- ½ lb pre-cooked pork belly
- 1 tomato
- ¼ balsamic vinegar
- 2 slices of your favorite bread

Directions:

1. Place the slices of bread in the toaster or under the oven broiler.
2. Slice the tomato into quarters.

3. Reheat your leftover pork belly in the microwave or oven so it is warm, but not hot.
4. Set a pan on the oven to medium heat and add oil. Once hot, place the tomato quarters in the pan and sear until their skins wrinkle from the heat.
5. To assemble the sandwich, layer the mozzarella slices, spinach, pork belly, and seared tomatoes on the toasted sandwich slices. The heated bread, pork, and tomatoes should begin to naturally melt the cheese. Drizzle everything with balsamic vinegar.
6. Enjoy!

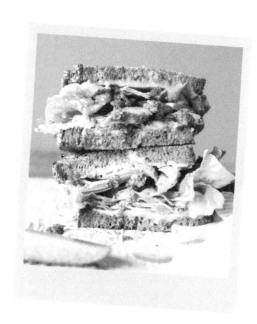

Shrimp and Avocado Bowl

Shrimp are a quick and easy way to pack in protein during lunch, plus they have all the vitamins and nutrients your body needs for boosting reproductive health. Combine this tiny but mighty shrimp with avocado and you have a delicious lunch that you'll want to repeat week after week.

Time: 15 minutes
Serving Size: 1
Prep Time: 5 minutes
Cook Time: 10 minutes
Nutritional Facts/Info:
1,388 calories, 52 g fat, 163 g protein, 76 g carbohydrates, 2 g sugar

Ingredients:

- 1 cup medium shrimp, detailed
- 1 avocado
- 1 serving quinoa
- 3 tbsp soy sauce
- 1 tsp salt
- 1 tsp paprika
- 1 tsp pepper

Directions:

1. Place a pot on the stove and add water per quinoa package directions. Cook per package directions.
2. While the quinoa is cooking, toss the thawed shrimp in a bowl with soy sauce, paprika, salt, and pepper.

3. Place a pan on the stove with a bit of olive oil. Once the pan is hot, add the seasoned shrimp to the pan. It should cook quickly, and it is finished when the color has changed from pale pink and white to a darker pink. Most shrimp is pre-cooked or boiled for safety.

4. Using a knife and a cutting board, slice the avocado in half. Remove the skin and the pit. Chop the avocado into cubes and season with salt and pepper.

5. To assemble, scoop the finished quinoa into a bowl. Top the quinoa with the shrimp and avocado.

6. Enjoy!

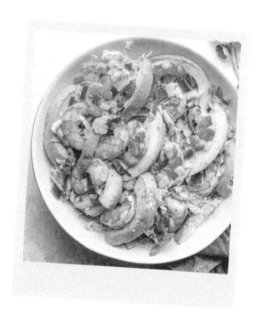

Sweet Potato and Black Bean Burrito Bowl

These vegetarian burrito bowls are great for soon-to-be parents who want to follow the fertility diet without giving up their other dietary needs. It is a great mix of sweet and savory, relies on plant-based proteins, and can serve two! This recipe is also easy to double, or even triple, for those who like to meal-prep their lunches.

Time: 55 minutes

Serving Size: 2

Prep Time: 15 minutes

Cook Time: 40 minutes

Nutritional Facts/Info: 473 calories, 2 g fat, 15 g protein, 96 g carbohydrates, 5 g sugar

Ingredients:

- 1 sweet potato
- 1 15 oz can black beans
- 1 cup rice
- 1 ½ cups chicken broth
- 1 tbsp cinnamon
- 2 tsp chili powder
- 2 tbsp lime juice
- 1 tsp salt
- 1 tbsp olive oil

Directions:

1. Preheat the oven to 375 °F.
2. Rinse the sweet potato, then using a knife and cutting board, chop the potato into one-inch cubes. You don't need to peel the skin.
3. Place the sweet potato cubes into a bowl. Drizzle the potatoes in olive oil and season with cinnamon, chili powder, and salt. Stir until thoroughly coated.
4. Arrange the sweet potatoes on a baking tray and bake them for 30 minutes.
5. Measure out the chicken broth and place it in a pot on the stove to boil. Then, add the rice to this mixture. It should cook exactly like a standard serving of rice, but the water has been substituted for chicken broth to give it extra flavor.
6. As the rice and sweet potatoes are cooking, open and drain the can of black beans. You can heat the beans on the stove or in the microwave, whichever is your preference. Set them aside.
7. When the sweet potatoes are done cooking, remove them from the oven.
8. Use a fork to fluff the rice and ensure all the liquid has been absorbed. Then, add the sweet potato pieces and the beans to the pot of rice. Stir until the ingredients are evenly distributed.
9. Drizzle lime juice over the mixture and serve in bowls.
10. Enjoy!

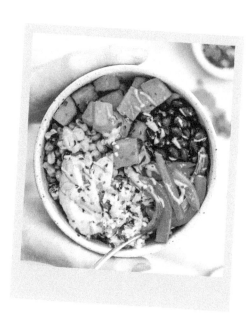

BLTA in a Bowl

BLT, otherwise known as a bacon, lettuce, and tomato sandwich, is getting a fertility friendly upgrade! Bacon, lettuce, tomato, avocado in a bowl are all of the healthy things you love about a BLTA but without the extra carbs. You can use a store purchased bottle of ranch dressing for this recipe or get creative and make your own. Either way, you will have a delicious and filling lunch to get you through the day.

Time: 30 minutes
Serving Size: 1
Prep Time: 10 minutes
Cook Time: 20 minutes
Nutritional Facts/Info:
755 calories, 64 g fat, 26 g protein, 25 g carbohydrates, 5 g sugar

Ingredients:

- 1 cup lettuce
- 1 tomato
- 3 strips bacon
- 1 avocado
- ¼ cup ranch dressing

Directions:

1. Preheat the oven to 350 °F.
2. Arrange your bacon on a baking sheet and place in the preheated oven to bake for 20 minutes.
3. While the bacon is cooking, slice the avocado in half. Remove the skin and the pits, then chop into one-inch cubes.

4. Similarly, chop the tomato into one-inch cubes, removing the stems.
5. Once the bacon is cooked, remove it from the oven and place the strips on a wire rack to cool for five minutes.
6. Using a knife or your hands, cut or break the bacon up into smaller pieces.
7. To assemble, place the lettuce in a bowl. Top with the chopped tomatoes, avocados, and bacon. Drizzle the entire thing with ranch dressing.
8. Enjoy!

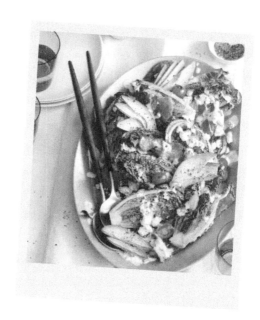

Quick Steak Curry

This recipe cuts down the typically long cook times of Indian food and reimagines it for a quick lunch. It also relies on fertility friendly foods like steak and whole-fat dairies. These foods are rich in protein and the nutrients that soon-to-be parents need for their reproductive health.

Time: 30 minutes

Serving Size: 2

Prep Time: 15 minutes

Cook Time: 15 minutes

Nutritional Facts/Info: 646 calories, 8 g fat, 56 g protein, 83 g carbohydrates, 6 g sugar

Ingredients:

- 1 filet of steak
- 4 tbsp whole-fat plain yogurt
- 1 tbsp chili powder
- 1 tbsp garam masala
- ½ tbsp ground coriander
- 2 tsp salt
- 1 cup rice
- ½ onion
- 1 red bell pepper
- ½ cup water

Directions:

1. Mix together the seasonings and yogurt in a bowl.
2. Using a knife and cutting board, slice the steak filet into long, thin strips. Add the strips to the bowl of yogurt and seasonings.
3. Mix the steak and seasonings until thoroughly combined.
4. Place a pot of water to boil on the stove and cook the rice per package instructions.
5. Chop the red pepper and onion into very small pieces, roughly ¼ inch in size.
6. Place a pan on the stove to medium heat and add the seasoned steak and vegetables in the pan. Cook for ten minutes, adding water halfway through. The water should boil off and create a thin sauce with the steak seasonings.
7. To assemble, add rice to your plate and ladle the meat and vegetables onto the rice.
8. Enjoy!

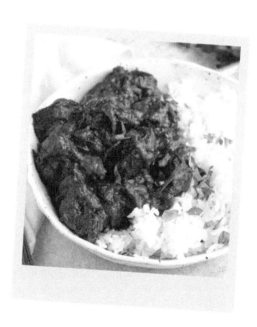

Beet Salad

Beets are a fantastic, fertility boosting food that you can easily incorporate into a rich salad. This salad is perfect for weekend lunches or a salad meal prep. It takes a bit longer to prepare, owing to the cook time of the beets, but patience pays off. Easily double or triple the ingredients to incorporate this salad into your weekly meal prep or enjoy the double serving listed below with your partner.

- Time: 80 minutes
- Serving Size: 2
- Prep Time: 20 minutes
- Cook Time: 60 minutes
- Nutritional Facts/Info:
  368 calories, 23 g fat, 16 g protein, 31 g carbohydrates, 14 g sugar

Salad Ingredients:

- 3 cups kale
- 3 beets
- ½ cup water
- ½ cup walnuts
- cup dried cranberries
- ¼ cup feta cheese

Dressing Ingredients:

- ¼ cup balsamic vinegar
- 3 tbsp olive oil
- 1 tsp brown mustard
- 1 tbsp honey

- 1 tbsp garlic
- 1 tsp salt

Directions:

1. Preheat the oven to 400 °F.
2. Arrange the beets on a baking tray with a ½ cup water and bake for one hour.
3. While the beets bake, make the salad dressing. Combine balsamic vinegar, olive oil, brown mustard, honey, garlic, and salt in a bowl. Whisk for two to three minutes or until fully combined.
4. Once cooked and soft, remove the beets from the oven. Allow them to cool, then peel away the skin using your fingers or a sharp knife.
5. Slice the peeled beets into small wedges and add the wedges to a bowl.
6. Cover the beets with half the dressing, the cooked beets will absorb the flavor from the dressing while you prepare the remainder of the salad.
7. In a separate bowl, add half the kale, walnuts, and dried cranberries. Toss until the ingredients are evenly distributed.
8. Top the salad with half of the seasoned beets and feta cheese.
9. Repeat steps seven and eight for the second salad.
10. Enjoy!

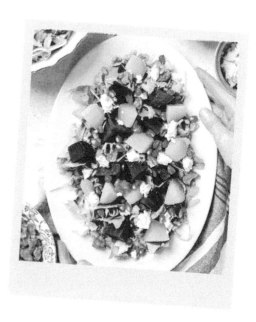

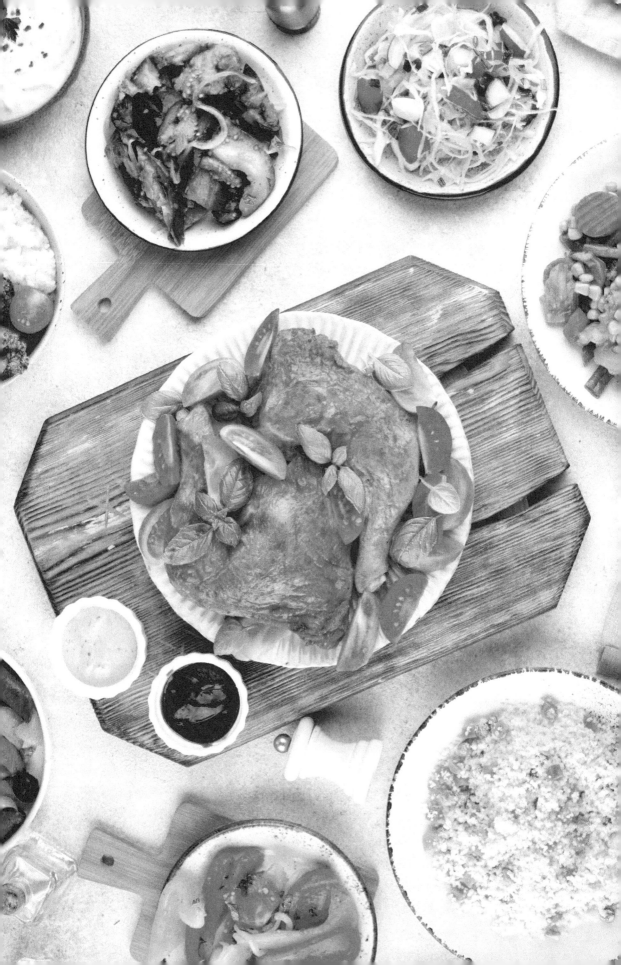

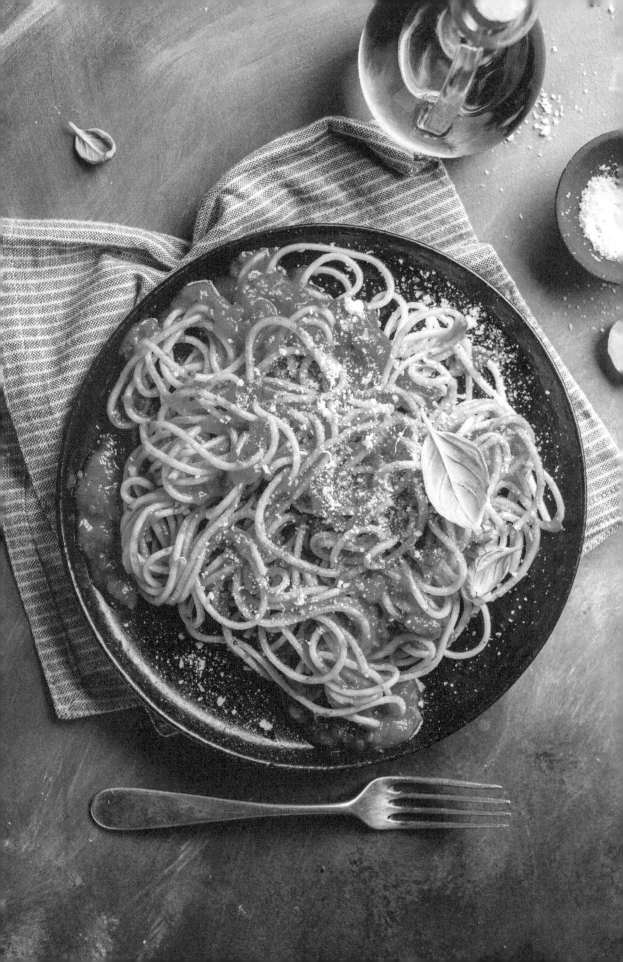

CHAPTER FIVE

Dinner

What's cooking? The options are endless! Dinner is a great time to get creative in the kitchen, and when following a fertility diet it is also the perfect time to pack in the fertility boosting vegetables and proteins that seem harder to incorporate into the other meals of the day. Taste test a few of my favorites like the turkey chili, grecian god bowl, and the sweet potato gnocchi. These recipes rely heavily on beef liver, oysters, spinach, salmon, and avocados, foods that are rich in hormone balancing nutrients, zinc, and estrogen. Some of these recipes create enough servings for entire families or dinner parties to enjoy a meal together. Little will your dinner guests know they are also having a fertility boost with their chili! Other recipes are geared towards smaller dinners for just the soon-to-be parents.

For best results, you'll want to make sure you have all the right tools in the kitchen. The most common tools required in these recipes are a cutting board, a sharp knife for cutting vegetables, a stock pot, scissors or screwdrivers for snapping oysters, and a food processor.

Pumpkin Power Salad

This fall-themed salad brings the basic salad to a new level. It is a great meal to share with family and friends while promoting your fertility. Pumpkin is a squash that helps balance hormones.

Time: 55 minutes

Serving Size: 4

Prep Time: 15 minutes

Cook Time: 40 minutes

Nutritional Facts/Info:

654 calories, 64 g fat, 14 g protein, 16 g carbohydrates, 2 g sugar

Salad Ingredients:

- 1 small pumpkin
- 1 cup rice
- 3 cups spinach
- 1 cup pecans
- 3 tbsp maple syrup or honey
- ¼ cup pomegranate seeds
- ¼ cup crumbled goat cheese
- Salt and pepper
- ¼ melted butter

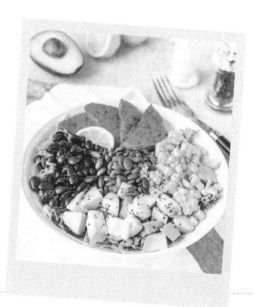

Dressing Ingredients:

- ½ cup tahini
- ¼ maple syrup or honey
- ¼ lemon juice

- ¼ olive oil
- 2 tbsp apple cider vinegar
- 2 tbsp minced garlic
- 1 tsp salt
- ¼ to ½ cup water

Directions:

1. Preheat the oven 425 °F.
2. Cut the pumpkin into slices, remove the seeds and spread on a baking sheet. Drizzle with melted butter, minced garlic, and salt.
3. Cook the pumpkin slices for 30 minutes, flipping halfway through.
4. Add the rice to a pot on the stove and cook per the box instructions.
5. While the rice cooks, add all of the dressing ingredients (tahini, maple syrup, lemon juice, olive oil, apple cider vinegar, salt, and proportionate amount of water) to a blender. Blend until smooth, adding water to make the mixture until your desired level of thinness. Set aside.
6. Place another pot on a burner at medium heat. Add pecans and maple syrup.
7. Caramelize the nut mixture for roughly five minutes.
8. Remove the pumpkin from the oven and let it cool for five to ten minutes.
9. Assemble the salad by adding spinach to a bowl, top with a few slices of pumpkin, caramelized nuts, and dressing.
10. Enjoy!

Speedy Salmon

Salmon is a must-eat for most fertility diets. This recipe allows soon-to-be parents to get all the benefits of salmon, without spending a long time in the kitchen. Get in, eat, and get out, so you can spend more time scheduling doctors appointments and preparing to expand the family.

Time: 20 minutes
Serving Size: 2
Prep Time: 5 minutes
Cook Time: 15 minutes
Nutritional Facts/Info:
569 calories, 29 g fat, 68 g protein, 13 g carbohydrates, 9 g sugar

Ingredients:

- 1 lb salmon
- 4 tbsp garlic
- 1 tbsp dijon mustard
- 1 tbsp butter
- 2 tbsp honey
- 1 tsp lemon juice
- ¼ tsp paprika
- tsp red pepper flakes (optional)
- Salt and pepper

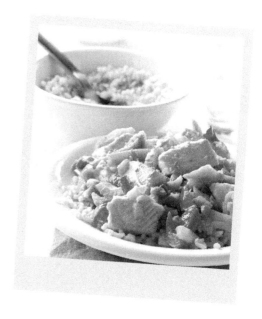

Directions:

1. Preheat the oven to 400 °F.
2. Place aluminum foil on a baking sheet, allow for excess, and place the salmon filet on top of the foil.
3. Mix together garlic, mustard, butter, lemon, honey, and seasonings in a separate bowl.
4. Pour the mixture on top of the salmon and bend the foil around the fish filet to keep the mixture from draining away from the fish.
5. Bake in the oven for 10 to 12 minutes.
6. Then, uncover the fish and switch the oven to the broiler setting.
7. Broil for two minutes until the crust just begins to brown.
8. Remove from the oven and serve warm. This dish is best served with another fertility boosting side vegetable, asparagus. See Chapter 7 for a tasty asparagus recipe.

Turkey Chili

This chili recipe is a crowd pleaser and a fertility wonder recipe. It is a time commitment to cook, but well worth the effort. Thanks to slow cookers and crock pots, you can add the ingredients to the pot and leave it to cook all day while you work and run errands. It is a fun recipe to put together with your spouse or friends. The seasonings, lean meat, and lentils in this recipe will promote fertility.

Time: 3 hours and 50 minutes
Serving Size: 6
Prep Time: 20 minutes
Cook Time: 3 hours and 30 minutes
Nutritional Facts/Info: 378 calories, 9 g fat, 30 g protein, 47 g carbohydrates, 4 g sugar

Ingredients:

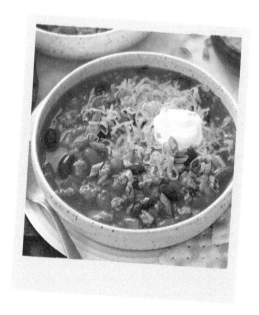

- 1 tbsp melted butter
- 1 lb ground turkey
- 1 tsp salt
- 1 tsp garlic powder
- 1 tsp pepper
- 1 tbsp chili powder
- 2 tsp cumin
- ½ tsp cinnamon
- ½ tsp turmeric
- ½ white onion
- ½ red bell pepper
- ¼ cup chipotle adobo peppers
- 2 sweet potatoes, cubed
- 1 cup quinoa
- 1 can black beans

- 28 oz can crushed tomato
- 4 cups beef broth
- 3 cups spinach
- 4 tbsp cilantro
- ¼ cup green onion

Directions:

1. Add butter to a skillet on medium to high heat.
2. Dice the onion, bell pepper, chipotle adobo peppers, and sweet potatoes
3. Once melted, add the onion to the pan. Cook for three to five minutes.
4. Add the ground turkey to the pan, cook for five minutes.
5. Transfer the mixture to a slow cooker, add the bell pepper, and season with salt, pepper, and garlic powder.
6. Add the sweet potatoes, broth, chipotle adobo peppers, quinoa, crushed tomatoes, and remaining seasonings to the pot.
7. Cook on high for three hours.
8. After three hours, stir in the spinach and allow to wilt.
9. Serve hot and top with cilantro and green onions.

Salmon Salad

This filling salmon salad will take any basic salad recipe to the next level. It is filled with fertility friendly vegetables and proteins. Turn this recipe into a sweet, stay-at-home date night with your partner. Pair it with any of the fantastic desserts from Chapter 7.

Time: 50 minutes

Serving Size: 2

Prep Time: 20 minutes

Cook Time: 30 minutes

Nutritional Facts/Info:

790 calories, 46 g fat, 17 g protein, 83 g carbohydrates, 1 g sugar

Salad Ingredients:

- 1 lb salmon
- 3 tbsp melted butter
- 2 tsp salt
- 2 tsp Italian seasoning
- 4 cups spinach
- ½ cup chopped broccoli
- 1 cup cooked brown rice
- 2 hard boiled eggs
- 1 avocado
- ¼ cup chopped walnuts

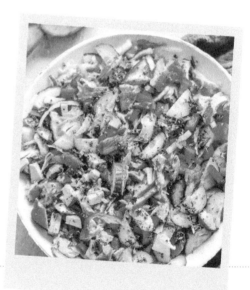

Dressing Ingredients:

- ¼ cup olive oil
- 1 tsp dijon mustard

- 2 tbsp red wine vinegar
- 1 tbsp lemon juice
- ¼ tsp minced garlic
- ½ tsp dried oregano
- Salt and pepper

Directions:

1. Preheat the oven to 350 °F.
2. Place salmon on a baking sheet and cover in melted butter, salt, and Italian seasoning.
3. Chop one ½ cup of broccoli florets and place around the baking sheet with the salmon.
4. Bake the salmon and broccoli for 1o to 12 minutes.
5. While the salmon bakes, place a pot of water to boil on the stove per the rice instructions. Cook until fluffy, per package instructions.
6. In one additional pot, boil water. Once the water reaches a roiling boil, add two eggs. Continue to boil for two minutes and then remove from the heat. Leave the eggs in the water for an additional seven minutes.
7. Remove the eggs from the hot water and immediately rinse in cold water. Peel the shells from the hard boiled eggs.
8. After the salmon, broccoli, eggs, and rice have finished cooking. Assemble the dressing while they cool. Combine all of the dressing ingredients in a bowl and whisk vigorously for two to three minutes.
9. Cut one avocado in half, remove the pit and skin. Then, slice the avocado into thin wedges.
10. To assemble the salads, place half of the spinach into one bowl and half into the other, it will create two salads. Layer on slices of salmon, rice, broccoli, hard boiled eggs, avocado, and walnuts. Drizzle with dressing to your choice.
11. Enjoy!

Oysters

It wouldn't be a fertility cookbook without recommending an oyster recipe. Oysters are the most effective fertility food; they are high in zinc.

Time: 50 minutes

Serving Size: 2

Prep Time: 30 minutes

Cook Time: 20 minutes

Nutritional Facts/Info:

725 calories, 58 g fat, 35 g protein, 17 g carbohydrates, 3 g sugar

Ingredients:

- 12 oysters
- 2 tbsp minced garlic
- 8 tbsp melted butter
- 1 tsp parsley
- ¼ tsp onion powder
- ¼ tsp black pepper
- 1 tbsp grated Parmesan cheese

Directions:

1. In a saucepan on the stove, melt butter over medium heat and add garlic. Cook until fragrant.
2. Remove from the heat and stir in the remaining seasonings, not including the cheese.
3. Place the butter mixture in the fridge until firm.
4. While the butter chills, rinse the oysters under cold water to remove any debris.

5. To crack open the oysters, find the flat end of a screwdriver, clean it thoroughly. Wedge the screwdriver into the 'hinge' of the oyster. Grab a sharp knife to cut the muscle and separate the top from the bottom of the oyster. Don't lose any of the liquid!

6. Preheat the oven to 400 °F.

7. Spoon the butter and Parmesan into each of the oysters.

8. Bake for 15 minutes and then switch to the broiler for two additional minutes.

9. Allow to cool for five minutes and serve warm!

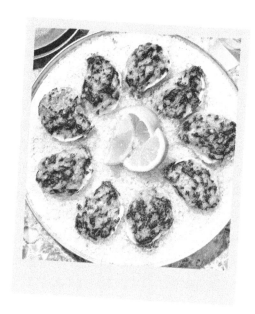

Beef Stuffed Avocados

Stuffed avocados will soon be your favorite low-carb dinner. They start with the perfect base for fertility health, avocados, which are rich in the healthy variety of fats that soon-to-be expecting mothers need for stronger ovulation. This recipe in particular relies on lean ground beef, and a 'taco' flavored stuffed avocado. It's your low-carb replacement for Taco Tuesday!

Time: 25 minutes
Serving Size: 2
Prep Time: 10 minutes
Cook Time: 15 minutes
Nutritional Facts/Info:
1,132 calories, 63 g fat, 91 g protein, 55 g carbohydrates, 6 g sugar

Ingredients:

- 2 avocados
- 1 lb lean ground beef
- 1 onion
- ½ cup shredded Monterey Jack cheese
- ½ cup chopped tomatoes
- ½ cup black beans
- 2 tbsp cumin
- 1 tbsp chili powder
- 1 tbsp garlic powder
- 2 tsp salt
- 1 tsp pepper

1. Cut each avocado in half and remove the pit. Then, using a spoon, scoop out some extra from the middle of the avocado to create a bowl. Set aside the excess avocado as you can use it for additional topping later.
2. Place a frying pan on the stovetop to medium heat and add the butter, allowing it to melt.
3. While the pan heats, chop one onion and slice the tomato into one-inch cubes.
4. Once heated, add the onion to the pan. Cook for three to five minutes before adding the ground beef.
5. Cook the onions and beef together until the beef begins to brown, then add the cumin, chili powder, garlic powder, salt, and pepper to the mixture.
6. When the meat mixture is seasoned thoroughly, add the beans and chopped tomatoes to the pan.
7. Spoon the filling from the pan directly into the hollowed out avocado. Top with cheese and serve hot!

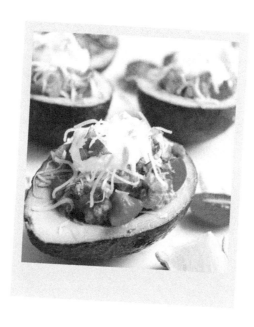

Vegetarian Stuffed Avocados

If beef isn't your favorite, but you still want to take advantage of the fertility filled nutritious dinner of a stuffed avocado, then consider assembling this meatless version. You can still get the great fertility benefits when you skip the meat and add a plant-based protein!

Time: 20 minutes

Serving Size: 2

Prep Time: 10 minutes

Cook Time: 10 minutes

Nutritional Facts/Info:

543 calories, 53 g fat, 31 g protein, 86 g carbohydrates, 16 g sugar

Ingredients:

- 2 avocados
- 1 can chickpeas
- 1 onion
- ½ cup shredded Swiss cheese
- ½ cup chopped tomatoes
- 2 tbsp lemon juice
- 1 tbsp garlic powder
- 2 tsp salt
- 1 tsp pepper

Directions:

1. Cut each avocado in half and remove the pit. Then, using a spoon, scoop out some extra from the middle of the avocado to create a bowl. Set aside the excess avocado as you can use it for additional topping later.

2. Place a frying pan on the stovetop to medium heat and add the butter, allowing it to melt.
3. While the pan heats, chop one onion and slice the tomato into one-inch cubes.
4. Once heated, add the onion to the pan. Cook for three to five minutes before adding the chickpeas.
5. Cook the onions and chickpeas together for three to five more minutes, then add the lemon juice, garlic powder, salt and pepper to the mixture.
6. When the meat mixture is seasoned thoroughly, add the chopped tomatoes to the pan.
7. Spoon the filling from the pan directly into the hollowed out avocado. Top with cheese and serve hot!

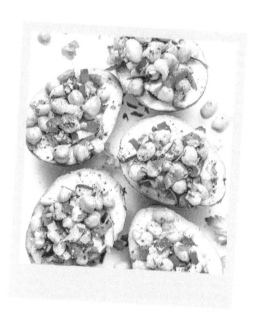

Salmon Wraps

Wraps are low-carb sandwiches that rely on tortillas rather than thick slices of bread. You can stuff wraps with any number of fertility boosting super-foods, including salmon. These are great for a quick weeknight dinner, and they can be made ahead of time for anyone who wants to incorporate fertility friendly ingredients into their meal prepping.

Time: 15 minutes

Serving Size: 2

Prep Time: 5 minutes

Cook Time: 10 minutes

Nutritional Facts/Info:

508 calories, 30 g fat, 20 g protein, 40 g carbohydrates, 3 g sugar

Ingredients:

- 1 salmon filet
- 2 spinach tortillas
- 1 cup spinach
- 4 tbsp vinegar
- ½ avocado
- 2 tbsp olive oil
- 2 tbsp lemon juice
- Salt and pepper

Directions:

1. Place a pan on the stove top at medium heat and drizzle with olive oil.
2. Season the salmon with salt, pepper, and lemon juice before placing it on the hot pan. Cook for five minutes, skin side down.

3. Flip the salmon to cook meat side down for an additional five minutes. Remove from heat and allow to cool.
4. Slice the avocado in half, remove the pit and the skin. Slice the avocado into strips.
5. Slice the salmon into bite-sized pieces or to your preference.
6. To assemble the wrap, place one tortilla flat on a plate top with half the spinach, avocado slices, salmon, and vinegar. Roll forward until it creates a long tube. Repeat for the second wrap.
7. Serve and enjoy with your favorite snacks and sides!

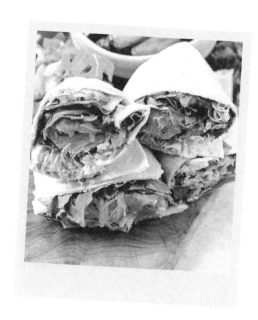

Beef Liver Kabobs

Liver is a fertility friendly meat that can scare off many amature cooks. However, there are easy and delicious ways to cook liver. You don't have to be an aspiring chef to serve this at a dinner party or even just dinner for two. This recipe is best cooked on an outdoor grill, but can be recreated inside with a skillet or cast iron pan.

Time: 45 minutes

Serving Size: 4

Prep Time: 35 minutes

Cook Time: 10 minutes

Nutritional Facts/Info:

672 calories, 22 g fat, 91 g protein, 22 g carbohydrates, 1 g sugar

Ingredients:

- 1 lb beef liver
- 2 jalapenos
- 3 tbsp garlic
- 1 tbsp paprika
- 3 tsp cumin
- 2 tbsp melted butter
- 1 tsp salt
- 1 tsp pepper
- 3 tbsp red wine vinegar

Directions:

1. Chop the liver into one-inch cubes.
2. In a bowl, mix together garlic, paprika, cumin, butter, salt, pepper, and red wine vinegar. Place the liver in the marinade and set aside for 30 minutes.

3. Preheat the grill to 425 °F or high heat.
4. Chop the jalapeno into discs, remove the seeds for a less spicy taste.
5. Rinse the kabob sticks in water to avoid charring and smoke.
6. Layer the marinated liver and jalapenos onto the kabob sticks in a repeating pattern. There should be enough for roughly eight kabobs.
7. Arrange the kabobs across the grill, and cook for 4 minutes on each side.
8. Remove from the heat and serve hot with your favorite backyard bbq side dishes.

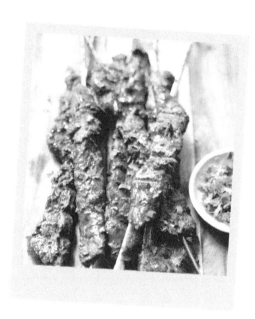

Chicken Liver Stir Fry

Another variety of liver that is good for fertility, chicken liver, can be easily used in place of chicken breasts and thighs in a stir fry dish. This can feed a crowd or make a sweet, date night meal. Liver is high in protein, vitamin A, and folic acid. The organ itself is a detoxifier, and basically the body's multivitamin. Three to four ounces of liver per week is recommended to pregnant women and those trying to conceive, so eat up!

Time: 25 minutes

Serving Size: 4

Prep Time: 10 minutes

Cook Time: 15 minutes

Nutritional Facts/Info:

415 calories, 15 g fat, 31 g protein, 35 g carbohydrates, 2 g sugar

Ingredients:

- 1 lb chicken liver
- 1 onion
- ½ cup water chestnuts
- 16 oz rice noodles
- 2 tbsp garlic
- ¼ soy sauce
- 2 tbsp olive oil
- ¼ rice vinegar
- Salt and pepper

1. Chop the chicken liver into bite-sized pieces and season with salt and pepper.
2. Add to a skillet on the stovetop and cook for 10 minutes, stirring occasionally to sear on all sides of the meat.
3. As the chicken liver cookes, slice the onion into rings and chop the water chestnuts in half.
4. Add rice noodles to a pot of boiling water, cook per package instructions.
5. Once the chicken liver is fully cooked, toss in the onions and water chestnuts. Saute until the onion has started to brown on the edges.
6. Ladle the rice noodles into the pan.
7. Drizzle soy sauce, rice vinegar, and garlic over the stirfry. Cook until fragrant.
8. Remove from heat and serve immediately.

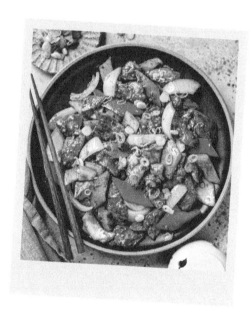

Grecian God Bowl

This rich and vegetarian-friendly fertility bowl embraces all the best Greek flavors. The Chickpeas in this meal are rich in protein and the vitamins and nutrients that soon-to-be parents need. Use a cast-iron skillet for best results.

Time: 1 hour and 15 minutes

Serving Size: 5

Prep Time: 15 minutes

Cook Time: 1 hour

Nutritional Facts/Info:

362 cal0ries, 62 g carbohydrates, 7 g fat, 17 g protein, 13 g sugar, 12 g fiber

Ingredients:

- 1 cup orzo
- 2 cups spinach
- 1 can chickpeas
- 1 onion
- 1 red bell pepper
- 12 oz can diced tomatoes
- 4 tbsp tomato paste
- 1 ½ cups vegetable stock
- 1 cup water
- 1 tbsp oregano
- 1 tsp red pepper flakes
- 1 tsp salt
- Feta

1. Dice and peel one onion into small pieces. Set aside.
2. Chop the red bell pepper into one-inch chunks and remove the seeds. Set aside.
3. Add the onion and the pepper to the pan and allow it to soften.
4. Add tomato paste to the veggies.
5. After five minutes, add the spinach, diced tomatoes, vegetable stock, water, and orzo. Bring to a simmer and allow to cook for 20 minutes.
6. Preheat the oven to 350°F.
7. After simmering, add the chickpeas, oregano, red pepper flakes, and salt.
8. Place the pan into the oven and cook for 30 minutes.
9. Remove from the oven and allow to cool for ten minutes.
10. Top with feta cheese and serve!

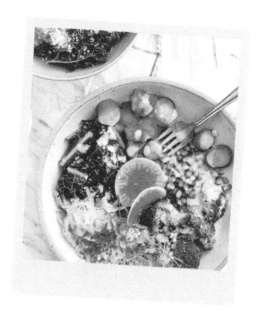

Roasted Pork Belly

Pork Belly is a cut of pork that is great for soon-to-be parents. It is rich in selenium, an antioxidant that promotes fertility in both men and women. Lucky for you, pork belly is also a crowd pleaser. It is great for backyard bbqs, dinners with family, and even just dinner for two. Enjoy this fertility friendly dinner with your favorite sides.

Time: 40 minutes

Serving Size: 4

Prep Time: 10 minutes

Cook Time: 30 minutes

Nutritional Facts/Info:

1,270 calories, 124 g fat, 18 g protein, 17 g carbohydrates, 13 g sugar

Ingredients:

- 1 lb pork belly
- ¼ cup soy sauce
- 1 orange
- 1 tbsp honey
- 2 tbsp brown sugar
- 1 tbsp white vinegar
- 2 tbsp minced garlic
- Salt and pepper

Directions:

1. Preheat the oven to 350 °F.
2. If not pre-cut, then use a knife to slice the pork belly into slices and score the fat.

3. Rub the pork belly with salt and place on a baking tray. Cook for 12 minutes before flipping the meat and cooking for another 12 minutes.
4. Switch the oven to the broiler, and continue to cook the pork under the broiler for three to five minutes.
5. While the meat is cooking, place a sauce pan on the stove top at low heat. Add the soy sauce, orange juice, honey, sugar, vinegar, and garlic.
6. Bring the sauce to a boil, stirring occasionally. Allow the sauce to cook for three to five minutes.
7. Remove the pork from the oven and arrange on a serving platter. Drizzle the meat with the sauce.
8. Serve hot and pair with a side of crispy asparagus from Chapter 7 for a full dinner. Enjoy!

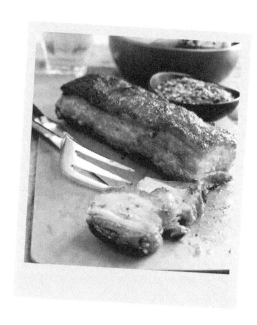

Pumpkin Curry

Don't let curries intimidate you. Anyone can cook a tasty curry, and with ingredients all found in a standard, American grocery store. The additions of steak and pumpkin, a hormone balancing superfood, to this dish make it a fertility boosting meal that is sure to please. Plus, it comes together in just under 45 minutes, easy for a weeknight dinner.

Time: 40 minutes

Serving Size: 4

Prep Time: 10 minutes

Cook Time: 30 minutes

Nutritional Facts/Info:

831 calories, 42 g fat, 32 g protein, 89 g carbohydrates, 23 g sugar

Ingredients:

- 2 tbsp olive oil
- 3 shallots
- 4 tbsp garlic
- 2 tbsp ginger
- 2 tbsp Thai red curry paste
- 6 cups chopped pumpkin
- 2 cans coconut milk
- ½ lb steak
- 2 tbsp lime juice
- 2 tbsp sugar
- 1 tsp salt
- 1 cup rice
- Cilantro and pumpkin seeds to garnish

1. Place a pot and a pan on the stove top at medium heat. Add the olive oil and allow it to heat up.
2. While the pot heats, chop the shallots into small pieces. Take this time to also cut the steak into one-inch slices.
3. Add the steak to the pan, cooking quickly to sear the sides but not cook all the way through. Remove from heat after one to two minutes on each side.
4. Add the shallots to the pot and cook for five to seven minutes, stirring often.
5. Once the shallots are turning translucent, add the garlic, ginger, and curry paste. Cook together for two to three minutes.
6. Pour the coconut milk into the mixture and stir until combined.
7. Add the pumpkin, steak, lime juice and sugar to the pot. Stir all the ingredients together and bring the pot back to a simmer. Cover the pot and allow it to cook for 10 to 15 minutes.
8. While the curry cooks, make one pot of rice per package instructions.
9. Remove the curry and rice from the heat. To assemble, spoon rice into bowls and top with the curry to your desired taste preferences.
10. Enjoy!

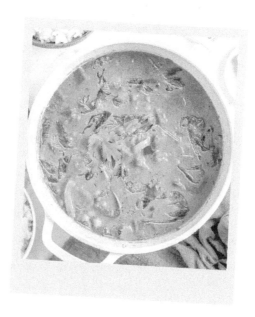

Oyster Stew

Want all the fertility benefits of oysters without eating oysters on the half shell? This stew is the perfect solution. The chunks of oyster meat, blend of seasonings, and rich sauce base make a great winter-time dinner. Or, enjoy this dish anytime you need comfort food or a taste of home. If you enjoy spicy foods, then feel free to substitute the green pepper for a jalapeno pepper to get that extra kick! Make this dish with either fresh or canned oysters, but remember if you are using fresh oysters that you'll need to account for the extra time it takes to shuck the oysters. If you opt for canned oysters, then add them to the soup when there is only two minutes left of the cooking process. The canned oysters cook much faster.

Time: 40 minutes
Serving Size: 6
Prep Time: 10 minutes
Cook Time: 30 minutes
Nutritional Facts/Info: 149 calories, 1 g fat, 4 g protein, 10 g carbohydrates, 5 g sugar

Ingredients:

- 4 tbsp butter
- 3 tbsp flour
- 1 onion
- 1 green bell pepper
- 1 stalk celery
- 1 tbsp cajun seasoning
- 2 cups milk
- ¼ oyster liquor, reserved from shucked oysters
- ¼ cup parsley

- ¼ cup green onions
- 4 tbsp garlic
- 24 oysters

Directions:

1. Mince the onion, and chop the green pepper, and celery into ½ inch bites.
2. Place a large pot on the stove over medium heat. Add the butter and cook until melted, then add the flour.
3. Stir the butter and flour constantly to create a roux. It should take about five minutes.
4. Add the vegetables to the pot and cook for two to three minutes.
5. Stir in the milk, oyster liquor, and cajun seasoning to the pot. Continue mixing until all the ingredients are evenly distributed.
6. Cook everything together for five minutes, this will allow all the flavors to get to know each other.
7. Add the parsley, green onion, garlic, hot sauce, and oysters to the pot. Cook for an additional five minutes. The edges of the oysters should curl when you approach five minutes.
8. Remove from heat and serve topped with oyster crackers or extra butter.

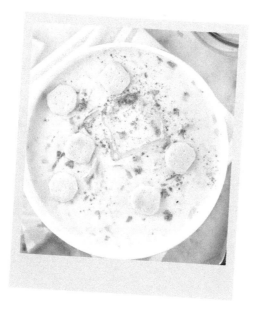

Fertility Casserole

Casseroles are typically comfort foods that remind us of home. They are simple to throw together, because they really are just a combination of several sides and main courses. In the case of this casserole, they can also be packed with healthy food choices. Many of the casseroles from childhood may be remembered as containing heavy pastas, five cheeses, and lots of cream cheese. Here, we've substituted the unhealthy ingredients for healthier ones and focused on the fertility boosting foods like chicken liver and chickpeas to balance your hormones and provide the vitamins and nutrients you need to follow a fertility diet.

Time: 55 minutes

Serving Size: 6

Prep Time: 10 minutes

Cook Time: 45 minutes

Nutritional Facts/Info:

458 calories, 14 g fat, 34 g protein, 47 g carbohydrates, 5 g sugar

Ingredients:

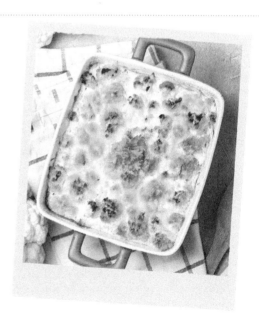

- 1 cup rice
- 1 can chickpeas
- ½ cup broccoli florets
- 1 lb chicken liver
- 2 cups chicken broth
- ¼ cup full fat Greek yogurt
- 1 cup shredded cheese
- 1 tsp salt
- ½ tsp pepper
- 2 tsp paprika

- 2 tsp garlic powder
- 1 tsp Italian seasoning

1. Add a pot of water to boil on the stove over medium heat. Place the slices of chicken liver into the pot to poach. Poaching the chicken, rather than cooking it in a frying pan, will stop it from drying out in the cooking process.
2. Cook the chicken liver for 10 to 12 minutes, rotating the chicken occasionally.
3. In another pot, cook the rice per package directions, using chicken broth instead of water. Any remaining chicken broth will be reserved for a later step.
4. Preheat the oven to 350 °F.
5. Chop the broccoli to remove the stems and the florets are bite-sized.
6. Remove the chicken liver from the heat and allow it to cool for a few minutes. Once cooled, slice the chicken liver into bite-sized pieces.
7. In a bowl, combine chicken liver, chickpeas, broccoli, 1 ½ cups cheese, yogurt, remaining chicken broth, and rice. Stir until the ingredients are fully combined. Add the seasonings and continue to stir.
8. Pour the mixture into a greased 9 x 13 casserole dish, top with the remaining cheese, and cover with tinfoil.
9. Place the casserole in the oven for 15 minutes, then remove the tinfoil and cook for an additional 10 minutes.
10. Remove from the oven and allow to cool for five minutes.
11. Enjoy!

Stuffed Chicken

These stuffed chicken breasts are a great alternative to another sheet pan of chicken and veggies. The Mediterranean flavors are delicious and nutritious, sure to impress at any dinner party or enhance a fun at-home date night. The vitamin A and folic acid in spinach is a fertility friendly food that really elevates this recipe along with the dairy and lean protein.

Time: 40 minutes

Serving Size: 4

Prep Time: 15 minutes

Cook Time: 25 minutes

Nutritional Facts/Info: 179 calories, 7 g fat, 24 g protein, 2 g carbohydrates, 1 g sugar

Ingredients:

- ½ cup feta cheese
- ½ cup red bell pepper
- ½ cup spinach
- ¼ cup kalamata olives
- 1 tbsp basil
- 1 tbsp parsley
- 3 tbsp minced garlic
- 4 chicken breasts
- 1 tbsp lemon juice
- 1 tbsp olive oil
- 1 tbsp Italian seasoning
- Salt and pepper

Directions:

1. Preheat the oven to 400 °F.
2. Using a cutting board and a sharpened knife, chop the red bell pepper into bite-sized pieces, chop the spinach and olives into similarly sized pieces. Remove the olive pits and spinach stems when chopping!
3. Combine the feta, peppers, spinach, olives, basil, parsley, and garlic in a bowl. Stir until well combined.
4. Cut a horizontal line through the thickest area of each chicken breast. Don't cut all the way through, you only need a pocket.
5. Season the chicken breasts with olive oil, Italian seasoning, salt, and pepper.
6. Scoop the filling into the pocket of each chicken breast. It should hold slightly more than a 1/4 cup. Use toothpicks to stabilize the chicken if necessary.
7. Arrange the chicken breasts on a baking tray and bake for 25 minutes.
8. Remove from the oven and drizzle with lemon juice.
9. Enjoy!

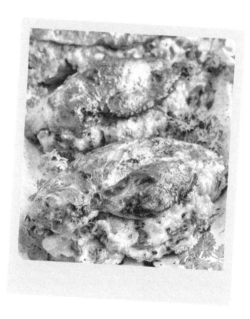

White Bean Chili

There's nothing better than a warm chili on a cool winter's evening, and this chili not only satisfies those cozy feelings, but follows the fertility diet as well. The plant based proteins found in this recipe will balance hormones and boost your fertility. While this dinner takes a bit longer to come together than some of the others in this book, it is worth the wait. Set those beans to cook on the stove, grab a book, and wait out the cook time.

Time: 1 hour and 30 minutes

Serving Size: 8

Prep Time: 15 minutes

Cook Time: 1 hour and 15 minutes

Nutritional Facts/Info: 218 calories, 4 g fat, 12 g protein, 35 g carbohydrates, 3 g sugar

Ingredients:

- 2 cups great northern beans
- 6 cups water
- 1 ½ cups chicken broth
- 1 onion
- 3 carrots
- 6 tbsp minced garlic
- 1 tbsp rosemary
- 2 tbsp olive oil
- Salt and pepper

Directions:

1. Place a large pot over medium heat on the stove top.
2. Add the beans, water, and salt to the pot. Allow to boil and then reduce to low heat. Simmer for one hour.
3. Once the beans are tender, drain them from the water. Reserve ½ cup of the liquid.
4. Pour ½ cup of the cooked beans and the reserved liquid into a bowl. Mash them together until they form a paste.
5. Using a cutting board and a knife, mince the onion and chop the carrots into one-inch cubes.
6. Return the pot to the stove and add olive oil. Once hot, place the minced onion and chopped carrots into the pot. Saute the vegetables until the carrots can be easily pierced with a fork, about five to seven minutes.
7. Stir in the garlic, rosemary, salt, pepper. Cook until fragrant or one to two minutes.
8. Add the mash beans, whole beans, and broth to the pot. Stir all the ingredients until well combined.
9. Bring the mixture to a boil and then reduce the heat to cook for five minutes.
10. Ladle into bowls and enjoy!

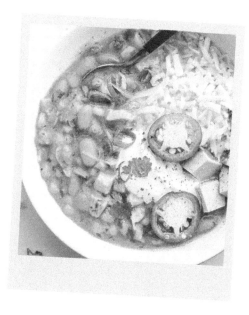

Spaghetti and Fertility Meatballs

Spaghetti and meatballs is a classic dish that can be easily adapted to the fertility diet. A few ingredient swaps and your Italian grandmother can expect many more grandchildren in the family tree. When purchasing the ground beef for the meatballs, be sure to find the version that includes organ meat, specifically liver. Ask the butcher's counter at the grocery store for assistance. Use this recipe when having friends or family over for a dinner party, or make it ahead of time for your weekly meal preps. Serve it up with your favorite sides. The options are endless!

Time: 50 minutes

Serving Size: 4

Prep Time: 10 minutes

Cook Time: 40 minutes

Nutritional Facts/Info:

918 calories, 38 g fat, 76 g protein, 82 g carbohydrates, 14 g sugar

Ingredients:

- 1 lb ground beef (including organs, liver)
- ½ cup bread crumbs
- 1 egg
- 1 package chickpea pasta
- 4 tomatoes
- 1 cup spinach
- 3 tbsp garlic
- 2 tbsp dried basil
- ¼ cup olive oil

- 1 tbsp butter
- 1 tsp red pepper flakes
- ¼ cup Parmesan

Directions:

1. In a bowl, combine the ground beef, bread crumbs, and egg. The mixture should come together like clay after a few minutes of kneading.
2. Shape the meat mixture into small balls, roughly 2 inches in diameter. There should be about 12 meatballs for this recipe, but you can easily double the ingredients if you need to make more. Place the meatballs on a tray and set in the freezer until you are ready to cook them.
3. Using a knife and cutting board, shop the four tomatoes into halves or quarters, remove the leaves and inner rind.
4. In a high-edged pan on the stove, melt the butter over medium heat.
5. Once melted, add the tomato chunks to the pan. Cook the tomatoes down, piercing occasionally with a wooden spoon for about five minutes. They should become very soft and mushy. You can remove the skins at this point or leave them in the sauce.
6. Place a pot of water on the stove and bring to a boil.
7. While waiting for the water to boil, add the garlic, basil, and olive oil to the simmering tomatoes. Stir the ingredients until they are evenly distributed.
8. Place the chickpea pasta into the boiling water, stir occasionally and cook per the box instructions.
9. Add the meatballs directly into the sauce and cover the pan with a lid for even cooking. Allow them to cook for five minutes before removing the lid and flipping the meatballs to brown the other side for about seven minutes.
10. Strain the pasta and set aside, reserving a ¼ cup of pasta water.
11. Once the meatballs are fully cooked stir in the pasta water and spinach to the sauce. Cook for roughly five minutes or until the spinach has wilted.
12. Optional: add the cooked pasta to the sauce pan and stir until the sauce has thoroughly coated all the noodles.

13. OR, if you prefer to control how much sauce is on each portion, spoon the noodles onto a plate and top with the sauce and meatballs.
14. Dust with Parmesan cheese and enjoy!

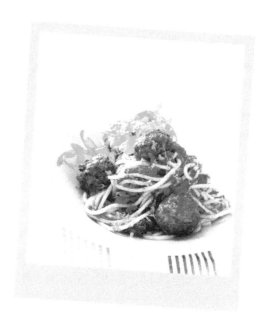

Loaded Pumpkin Bake

A fertility friendly take on the loaded baked potato skins, this recipe is great for family style dining. Slice into the delicious pumpkin and pass around the table. This recipe relies on the hormone balancing powers of pumpkin, the vitamin A and folic acid found in spinach, and other fertility superfoods like walnuts.

Time: 42 minutes

Serving Size: 4

Prep Time: 10 minutes

Cook Time: 32 minutes

Nutritional Facts/Info: 577 calories, 19 g fat, 92 g protein, 7 g carbohydrates, 2 g sugar

Ingredients:

- 1 pumpkin
- 2 cups spinach
- ¼ cup walnuts
- 1 cup shredded pork
- ¼ cup crumbled feta
- 2 tbsp olive oil
- Salt and pepper

Directions:

1. Preheat the oven to 425 °F.
2. Cut the pumpkin in half, removing any seeds and stems. Drizzle it in olive oil and place face down on a baking tray.
3. Bake the pumpkin for 20 minutes, flipping halfway for an even bake.
4. Remove the pumpkin from the oven.

5. In a bowl combine the spinach, shredded pork, walnuts, salt, and pepper. You can purchase pre-cooked and shredded pork from most grocery stores or your favorite local BBQ restaurant. If you'd prefer to cook and shred the pork yourself, then refer to the recipe for Roasted Pork Belly and shred that home-cooked pork with two grilling forks.

6. Spoon the mixture into the baked pumpkin and return to the oven for ten minutes. Once cooked, switch to the broiler for an additional two minutes.

7. Remove from the oven and sprinkle with the crumbled feta cheese.

8. Enjoy!

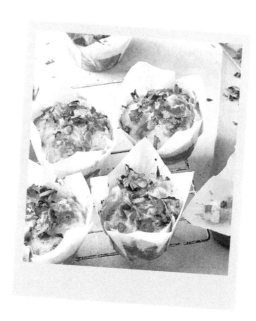

Falafel

Falafel is a popular Greek street food made with fertility boosting chickpeas. It is an adventurous dinner to make it home that is sure to satisfy your cravings, while boosting your fertility. This meal is easy to turn into a fun date night at home! Add in some extra Greek sides, throw on a movie, and indulge while knowing you are following your diet. To make falafel extra filling, use pita bread to create a falafel sandwich.

Time: 55 minutes

Serving Size: 2

Prep Time: 45 minutes

Cook Time: 10 minutes

Nutritional Facts/Info:

709 calories, 36 g fat, 25 g protein, 74 g carbohydrates, 12 g sugar

Ingredients:

- 1 can chickpeas
- ½ red onion
- ½ cup parsley
- 2 tbsp flour
- 2 tbsp olive oil
- ¼ cup tahini sauce

OPTIONAL

- 1 cup spinach
- 2 pita bread slices

1. Mince half of one red onion.
2. Place the red onion, parsley, flour, and chickpeas into a food processor. Blend until they form a sticky paste.
3. Using your hands, form the mixture into two-inch discs. They should be flat, not like spheres. Arrange the discs on a tray and place in the freezer for 30 minutes. The longer you can freeze them ahead of time, the better they will hold together when cooking.
4. Once firm, remove from the freezer. Place a pan over a burner on high and add olive oil to the pan.
5. Add the frozen falafel to the pan and cook for five minutes. Then, using tongs, flip the falafel discs to cook the other side for an additional five minutes or until the surface has turned brown and crunchy.
6. Remove the cooked falafel from the pan and place them on a wire rack to drain and cool.
7. Serve with tahini sauce for dipping, or assemble falafel sandwiches with the pita bread and spinach. Use the tahini sauce as a delicious condiment.
8. Enjoy!

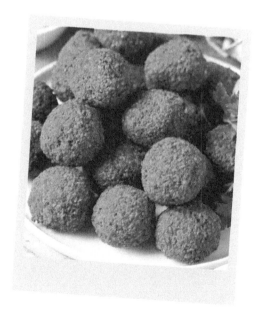

Beef Liver Tacos

It's the taco Tuesday of your fertility diet! Tacos are a simple dinner recipe that come together in a matter of minutes. They are customizable, and best of all, most of the ingredients are easy to swap out for fertility friendly alternatives.

Time: 25 minutes
Serving Size: 4
Prep Time: 10 minutes
Cook Time: 15 minutes
Nutritional Facts/Info:
541 calories, 27 g fat, 35 g protein, 38 g carbohydrates, 1 g sugar

Ingredients:

- 8 soft, corn tortillas
- 1 lb beef liver
- ½ cup shredded quesadilla cheese
- 2 avocados
- ½ an onion
- 1 lime
- 1 tsp salt
- 2 tbsp chili powder
- 2 tbsp cumin
- 1 tsp garlic powder
- 2 tbsp olive oil

1. Using a sharp knife, cut the filet of beef liver into strips. Make sure these strips are just smaller than the size of your tortillas.

2. In a bowl, combine the beef liver strips with the salt, chili powder, cumin, garlic powder, and olive oil. Stir the meat until the seasonings are evenly spread across all the pieces.

3. Place a skillet on the stove set to medium heat. Once warm, add the meat to the skillet. Cook for 7 minutes, turning occasionally to sear all sides.

4. While the meat cooks, chop half of an onion into small pieces.

5. Slice the avocado in half, remove the skin and the pit. Slice or chop the avocado into slices per your preference.

6. When the meat is done cooking, remove from the heat and set aside. With the pan still hot, place two tortillas at a time, face down, in the leftover juice from the meat. Toast the tortillas lightly for two minutes. Repeat for all remaining tortillas.

7. To assemble the tacos, place a toasted tortilla on a plate. Top the tortilla with cheese, then the meat, then the onion and avocado. Squeeze lime juice onto the assembled taco for a fresh taste.

8. Enjoy!

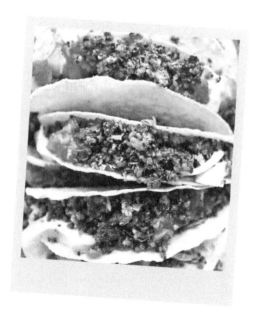

Cheesy Beet Pasta

This pasta is sure to impress at any dinner party. It is great for fertility thanks to the contribution of the hormone balancing beets plus the chickpea based pasta. Even better? It is hot pink! The roasted beets will become a dark magenta when cooked and mixed with the cheese and noodles; it is a very fun way to serve a meal. Beets are a recently researched fertility superfood that balances hormones and improves reproductive health in men and women.

Time: 70 minutes

Serving Size: 4

Prep Time: 10 minutes

Cook Time: 60 minutes

Nutritional Info: 750 calories, 35 g fat, 52 g protein, 75 g carbohydrates, 16 g sugar

Ingredients:

- 3 beets
- 3 cloves garlic
- ¼ cup olive oil
- 1 box chickpea pasta
- 1 cup Parmesan
- ¼ cup dried basil
- 2 tbsp sun dried tomato oil

Directions:

1. Preheat the oven to 400 °F.
2. Rinse the beets and peel the skin from them with a peeler or paring knife.

3. Wrap the peeled beets in tin foil. Arrange them with the cloves of garlic and drizzle in olive oil. Bake the package for 45 minutes.
4. While the beets roast, cook the chickpea pasta per package instructions.
5. When you remove the beets from the oven they should be soft to the touch and fragrant.
6. Place the whole contents of the tinfoil wrap into a blender and blend until smooth.
7. Transfer the blended beets to a pan over medium heat. Slowly add the Parmesan cheese, dried basil, and sun dried tomato oil. Stir until the cheese has melted completely, roughly five minutes.
8. Pour the cooked pasta into the pan and coat it thoroughly in the sauce. Cook the pasta in the sauce for an additional two to three minutes.
9. Remove the heat and serve!

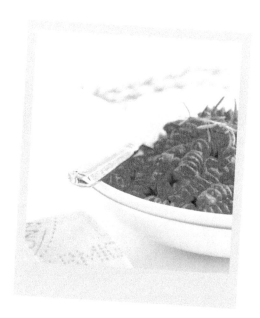

Oyster Casserole

If you would rather work with canned oysters than fresh oysters, this is the recipe for you. Get all the fertility boosting powers of oysters in a simple and cheesy casserole that everyone can enjoy. This recipe is also packed with vegetables to make a nutritious and well-rounded dinner. When making the rue, make sure to stir continuously to avoid the milk becoming grainy. A rue that is constantly stirred on a low temperature will stay silky smooth.

Time: 60 minutes

Serving Size: 4

Prep Time: 15 minutes

Cook Time: 45 minutes

Nutritional Facts/Info:

655 calories, 46 g fat, 25 g protein, 37 g carbohydrates, 5 g sugar

Ingredients:

- ½ onion
- 1 green bell pepper
- 1 stalk celery
- ¼ cup minced scallions
- 3 tbsp garlic
- Two 16 0z cans oysters
- 1 cup mushrooms
- ½ cup heavy cream
- ¼ cup Parmesan cheese
- 1 cup bread crumbs
- 2 tbsp olive oil
- ½ cup butter (1 stick)

- 2 tbsp flour
- 1 tbsp lemon juice
- 1 tbsp Worcestershire sauce
- 1 tsp salt

Directions:

1. Preheat the oven to 400 °F.
2. Using a cutting board and sharp knife, mince half the onion into tiny pieces and mince the shallot until you have reached ¼ cup. Then, chop the celery and green pepper into roughly one-inch pieces. Save the leftover onion and shallot for a future dinner.
3. Place a pan on the stove to medium heat and add 2 tbsp of the butter. Once the butter has melted, place the onion, pepper, and celery into the pan. Cook the vegetables together for five minutes. Then, add the shallots and garlic to the pan and cook for an additional two minutes.
4. Open the cans of oysters and drain them so there is very little liquid left in the can. Dump the drained oysters into the pan along with the mushrooms. Simmer the ingredients for five additional minutes.
5. Remove the pan from the heat.
6. In a separate pan over low heat, melt an additional 2 tbsp of butter. Once melted, add the flour to the pan. Whisk the ingredients together until they are smooth and bubbling. It should take one to two minutes.
7. Pour in the heavy cream to the pan and stir continuously for three to four minutes. To avoid the milk becoming grainy, do not stop stirring.
8. Add lemon juice, worcestershire sauce, and salt to the rue. Keep stirring for five minutes or until the sauce is simmering.
9. Once simmering actively, add the Parmesan cheese to the rue. Continue to stir while the cheese melts, roughly three minutes. Lower the heat until the burner is barely turned on.
10. Return to the pan of oysters and veggies. Using a mesh strainer or colander, drain the contents of the pan so that no liquid remains. Then, add the drained oysters and

vegetables to the cheese sauce. Mix until the ingredients are evenly distributed.

11. Pour the mixture into an 11 x 7 inch baking tray.

12. Place the remaining butter in a microwave safe dish and microwave for 30 seconds or until it has melted.

13. Toss the melted butter with the bread crumbs and spread the mixture across the top of the casserole.

14. Bake for 15 minutes and then broil for two minutes.

15. Serve hot and enjoy!

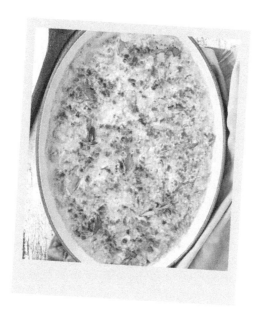

Sweet Potato Gnocchi

Gnocchi is a fun and creative way to get your pasta fix. You can swap out the flour in this recipe for your favorite gluten free alternative if you want to reduce the carbohydrates as much as possible. This recipe is more of a project, but it can make a fun date night recipe to make with your partner while improving your fertility health.

Time: 60 minutes

Servings: 2

Prep Time: 15 minutes

Cook Time: 45 minutes

Nutritional Facts/Info:

887 calories, 58 g fat, 46 g protein, 53 g carbohydrates, 4 g sugar

Ingredients:

- 1 sweet potato
- ¾ cup flour
- 1 tsp salt
- 1 egg
- ¼ cup olive oil
- 2 cup spinach
- ½ cup Parmesan
- 1 tbsp butter

Directions

1. Preheat the oven to 375 °F.
2. Pierce the sweet potato with a fork in eight to ten places, then place on a baking tray and bake for 30 minutes.

3. Once the potato is soft, remove from the oven. Peel away the skin of the sweet potato and add the meat of the sweet potato to a bowl.
4. Mash the sweet potato until smooth. Add the egg and stir until it is incorporated fully.
5. Slowly add the flour to the sweet potato mixture. It should come together in a stiff dough. Dump the mixture onto the counter to knead and do so for three to five minutes. Wrap in plastic wrap and allow to rest for 15 minutes.
6. Once rested, cut the mass of dough into four even sections. Roll each section into a long, thin rope. Using a knife, cut the long rope into one-inch sections.
7. Place a pot of water to boil on the stove with salt.
8. Once boiling, dump the gnocchi into the water and cook for two minutes or until the potato pasta cubes begin to float. Strain them in a colander.
9. Place a pan on the stove to medium heat. Add the butter to the pan and allow it to melt. When the butter has melted, add the spinach to the pan. Cook the spinach for three minutes.
10. Add the cooked gnocchi to the pan of spinach. Cook for five more minutes, this should sear the sides of the pasta.
11. Stir in the olive oil and Parmesan to the gnocchi and spinach. The Parmesan should just begin to melt so your scoop of pasta has a satisfying cheese pull.
12. Serve hot and enjoy!

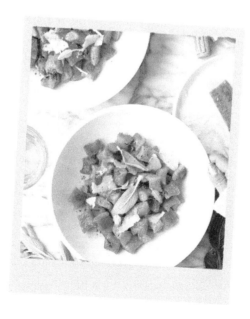

Garlic Butter Salmon

This salmon is tasty and perfectly follows your fertility diet. It is best served with a side of asparagus or leafy greens. Check out chapter seven for some great side dish recipes to accompany this dish. It comes together quickly, makes a romantic date night meal, and can be easily doubled if you are serving more than two.

Time: 15 minutes

Serving Size: 2

Prep Time: 3 minutes

Cook Time: 12 minutes

Nutritional Facts/Info: 342 calories, 30 g fat, 14 g protein, 5 g carbohydrates, 0 g sugar

Ingredients:

- 1 salmon filet
- 5 tbsp butter
- 4 tbsp minced garlic
- 1 tbsp olive oil
- 1 tsp salt
- 1 tsp dried basil

Directions:

1. Preheat the oven to 375 °F.
2. Place the butter in a microwave safe dish and microwave for 10 seconds or until the butter is just softened, not melted.
3. Stir in the garlic, olive oil, salt, and dried basil to the softened butter.
4. Spread the butter mixture across the pink meat of the salmon.

5. Place the seasoned salmon on a baking dish and bake for 12 minutes.

6. Remove from the oven and allow to cool for a few minutes.

7. Serve warm and enjoy!

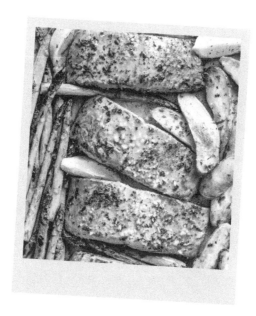

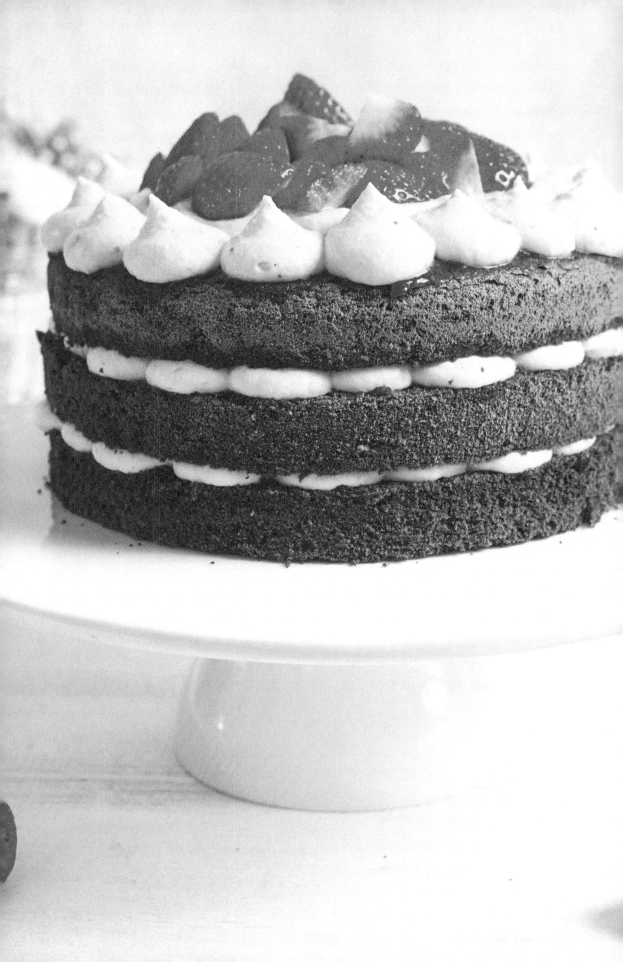

CHAPTER SIX

Desserts

You can satisfy your sweet tooth and follow a fertility diet at the same time. Yes, there are even dessert recipes that can boost reproductive health and balance hormones. Taste test a few of my favorites like the chocolate bark, sweet protein bites, and sweet potato bread. These recipes rely on pumpkin, avocado, walnuts, and sweet potatoes. Nutrients like zinc, iron, and fatty acids are strengthening eggs, semen, and overall fertility. No matter which dessert is your favorite, those that rely on chocolate, fruit, or creams, you can find a recipe below that works for you. These dishes will please a crowd, so bring one to your next party or office event too. Desserts that follow the fertility diet can still be enjoyed by everyone, not just soon-to-be parents.

For best results, you'll want to make sure you have all the right tools in the kitchen. The most common tools required in these recipes are baking dishes, parchment paper, electric mixers, and freezers.

Sweet Potato Cheesecake

This delicious dessert combines the fertility power houses of nuts and sweet potatoes for a sweet treat that will balance your hormones and boost your fertility while appeasing your sweet tooth. It is a great dessert to experiment with in the kitchen, turn it into a stay-at-home date night with your spouse!

An important note, make sure to make this recipe with coconut cream, not coconut milk. There is a difference, but both should be available in your local grocery stores.

Time: 2 hours

Serving Size: 8

Prep Time: 90 minutes

Cook Time: 30 minutes

Nutritional Facts/Info:

1,070 calories, 83 g fat, 16 g protein, 79 g carbohydrates, 53 g sugar

Crust Ingredients:

- 1 ½ cups pecans
- 1 cup chopped dates
- ¼ tsp salt

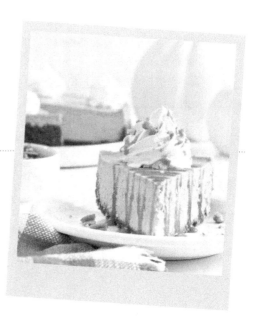

Filling Ingredients:

- 13 oz can coconut cream
- 2 cups raw cashews
- ½ cup maple syrup
- ¼ cup lemon juice
- 2 tsp vanilla

- 1 sweet potato
- 2 tbsp maple syrup
- 2 tsp pumpkin pie spice

Directions:

1. To make the crust, add pecans, chopped dates, and salt to a food processor. Blend until it forms a dough.
2. Press the dough into the bottom of a pie tin or baking dish. Store in the freezer until the filing is ready.
3. To begin the filling, preheat the oven to 375 °F.
4. Chop one sweet potato into one-inch squares. Season with salt and melted butter. Spread across a baking sheet and bake for 30 minutes or until soft.
5. Place the baked sweet potato cubes in a food processor and blend until creamy. Scoop out into a bowl and set aside.
6. Add again to a food processor, coconut cream, cashews, maple syrup, lemon juice, and vanilla. Blend until smooth.
7. Remove half of the mixture from the food processor, but leave the other half in the food processor. Continue to add the pureed sweet potato back along with the remaining maple syrup and seasonings. Blend until incorporated.
8. Retrieve the freezing crust and spread the half of the filling that was held back from the food processor. Smooth it and place back in the freezer for 15 to 20 minutes to set.
9. Once set, remove from the freezer and add the next layer of filling, the one that contains the pureed sweet potato. Smooth the filing over and put back in the freezer for another 30 minutes or until ready to serve.

Brownies

This unique brownie recipe doesn't contain traditional brownie ingredients, but you can't taste the difference. Indulge without guilt! Make these for a weeknight treat or enjoy an evening of experimentation with your partner in the kitchen. Cooking can bring people together, so make it a sweet date night and work towards your goal of parenthood.

Time: 35 minutes

Serving Size: 24

Prep Time: 20 minutes

Cook Time: 15 minutes

Nutritional Facts/Info: 99 calories, 3 g fat, 4 g protein, 16 g carbohydrates, 5 g sugar

Ingredients:

- 1 ¾ cup adzuki beans
- ¾ cup cocoa powder
- ¼ cup honey
- ¼ cup maple syrup
- 2 tbsp ground flaxseed
- 5 tbsp warm water
- 3 tbsp coconut oil
- 1 tsp salt
- 1 tsp vanilla
- 1 ½ tsp baking powder
- ½ tsp cinnamon
- ¼ cup walnuts

1. Preheat the oven to 325 °F.
2. Rinse and drain the adzuki beans, if you aren't using precooked beans then take this time to cook the beans per package instructions.
3. In the bowl of a stand mixer, combine water and flaxseed. Let those ingredients rest for five minutes.
4. Add coconut oil, honey, maple syrup, cocoa powder, salt, vanilla, baking powder, cinnamon, and cooked beans to the bowl. Mix on a medium speed for three minutes or until the batter has become thick.
5. Grease a mini muffin tin and divide the batter evenly amongst the slots. Add a few walnuts to each brownie.
6. Bake for 12 to 15 minutes.
7. Remove from the oven and allow the brownies to cool for ten minutes before enjoying your first bite.

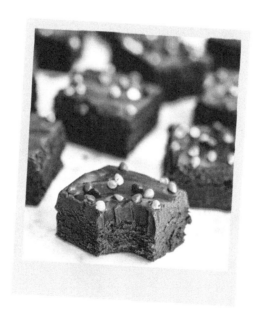

Berry Cheesecake

Fruity desserts are a guaranteed way to satisfy your sweet tooth while following your fertility diet. This cheesecake relies on low Glycemic Index fruits to boost fertility; as well as, using whole-fat dairy to create that classic cheesecake filling. Cheesecake is easiest to bake when using a springform pan which can be purchased from any major home-goods retailer or online.

Time: 105 minutes

Serving Size: 8

Prep Time: 30 minutes

Cook Time: 75 minutes

Nutritional Facts/Info:

741 calories, 56 g fat, 13 g protein, 51 g carbohydrates, 40 g sugar

Filling Ingredients:

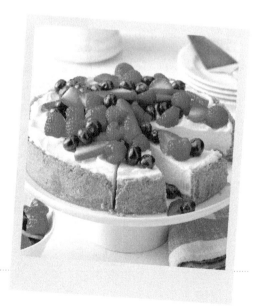

- 32 oz cream cheese
- 1 cup of sugar
- cup whole-fat Greek yogurt
- 1 ½ tsp vanilla extract
- 4 eggs
- ½ cup blueberries
- ½ cup raspberries
- 2 tbsp honey

Crust Ingredients:

- 1 ½ cups crushed Graham crackers
- 2 tbsp sugar

- 1 tbsp brown sugar
- ½ cup butter melted

Directions:

1. Begin by making the crust. Add graham crackers to a sealed plastic bag and crush by hitting the bag with a rolling pin or your fist. Continue until you have created 1 ½ cups of crushed cracker.
2. In a bowl, combine the crushed graham cracker with all the remaining crust ingredients. Stir well.
3. Press the wet crust into the bottom of a springform pan and set aside.
4. To create the filling, add the cream cheese to the bowl of a stand mixer and whip for two to three minutes.
5. Add the sugar and continue mixing until smooth, then stir in the yogurt and vanilla.
6. Once those ingredients are thoroughly mixed, whisk four eggs in a separate bowl. Return the mixer to a slow speed and slowly pour in the whisked eggs, one at a time until completely incorporated. Use a spatula to scrape the sides of the bowl if necessary.
7. Preheat the oven to 325 °F.
8. Pour the filing over top of the crust in the springform pan. Even out any lumps.
9. Bake for 75 minutes.
10. While the cheesecake bakes, place a pot on the stove top set to medium/low heat.
11. Add the blueberries, raspberries, and honey to the pan. Stir and mash until the fruit has turned into a compote. There should be a few whole pieces remaining in the mixture.
12. Remove the cheesecake from the oven and let it cool for 15 minutes before releasing the springform pan. You should be left with a perfectly round cheesecake.
13. Pour the fruit compote mixture over the cheesecake, garnishing with additional fresh fruit to your taste.
14. Place the whole cake in the fridge to chill for an hour and enjoy cold.

Watermelon Sorbet

This chilly, summertime treat is a great addition to any backyard barbeque. Watermelons contain a high level of glutathione, which is good for increasing the quality of a woman's eggs. Satisfy your sweet tooth, cool off, and give your fertility a boost, all at the same time.

Time: 4 hours and 20 minutes
Serving Size: 4
Prep Time: 20 minutes
Cook Time: 4 hours
Nutritional Facts/Info: 128 calories, 0 g fat, 1 g protein, 34 g carbohydrates, 32 g sugar

Ingredients:

- 3 cups watermelon
- ½ cup water
- ½ cup sugar
- 1 tsp lemon juice

Directions:

1. Place a pot of water to boil on the stove. Add sugar and lemon juice to the sizzling water. Stir it until fully dissolved.
2. Remove from heat once boiling and allow to cool to room temperature.
3. Chop three cups worth of watermelon, removing seeds if necessary, and place in a food processor. Add the cooled water mixture.

4. Blend the watermelon mixture for one to two minutes.

5. Pour the slushy into a 9 x 13 baking dish and freeze for three to four hours or overnight.

6. Enjoy!

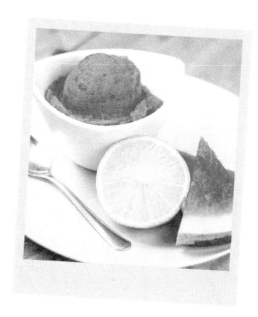

Nut Cake

This fall flavored nut cake is packed with the rich, plant-based proteins and complex carbohydrates that are ideal for soon-to-be parents. Remember, cake is even better when shared with friends. Bundt cakes can comfortably be cut into eight even slices.

Time: 60 minutes

Serving Size: 8

Prep Time: 20 minutes

Cook Time: 40 minutes

Nutritional Facts/Info:

351 calories, 15 g fat, 7 g protein, 50 g carbohydrates, 25 g sugar

Ingredients:

- ½ cup dark chocolate chips
- ½ cup chopped walnuts
- 1 cup flour
- 4 bananas
- ¾ cup brown sugar
- 2 eggs
- ¼ cup vegetable oil
- ¾ cups rolled oats
- 1 tsp baking powder
- 1 tsp baking soda
- ½ tsp salt
- 1 tsp cinnamon

1. Preheat the oven to 325 °F.

2. Peel the bananas and add them to a bowl. Mash the bananas with a fork until no lumps remain.

3. Add brown sugar, eggs, and oil to the bowl. Mix until the ingredients are fully incorporated.

4. In a separate bowl, combine flour, oats, baking powder, baking soda, salt, and cinnamon. Once fully combined, add these ingredients to the bowl of wet ingredients.

5. Mix the wet and dry ingredients together. Once mixed, add in the chocolate chips and chopped walnuts.

6. Grease a bundt pan.

7. Pour the batter into the bundt pan and place in the preheated oven. Bake for 40 minutes.

8. Once baked, remove the cake from the oven and let it cool fully before flipping from the pan.

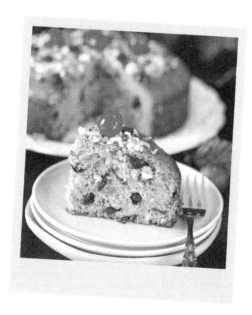

Pumpkin Pie

This traditional Thanksgiving dessert is secretly great for fertility! Pumpkins are a superfood that balances hormones. When you take the extra effort of making pumpkin pie fresh from a baking pumpkin, you are taking advantage of countless extra health benefits. Enjoy this holiday dish anytime and indulge without any guilt.

Time: 50 minutes

Serving Size: 8

Prep Time: 50 minutes

Cook Time: Varies

Nutritional Facts/Info: 187 calories, 9 g fat, 3 g protein, 24 g carbohydrates, 14 g sugar

Ingredients:

- 1 pumpkin
- 1 pie crust
- 2 tsp cinnamon
- 2 tsp all-spice
- ½ tsp nutmeg
- 1 tsp pumpkin pie spice
- ½ cup evaporated milk
- 1 egg

Directions:

1. Preheat the oven to 350 °F.
2. Cut the pumpkin in half, and cut off the stem, and place it on a baking tray with the meat side facing up.

3. Bake the pumpkin for 40 minutes.

4. Remove the pumpkin from the oven. Once cooled, place the pumpkin halves in a bowl and mash them until smooth.

5. Add the spices, evaporated milk, and egg to the mashed pumpkin. Mix thoroughly until it has a smooth consistency.

6. If the pie crusts require any pre-baking, then bake them according to package directions. If they do not require pre-baking, then pour the pumpkin mixture into the shell. Bake per package instructions.

7. Enjoy warm or chilled!

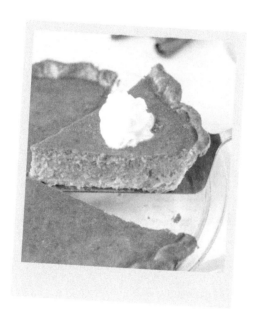

Banana Pudding

Pudding is a simple dish to serve for a tasty dessert that serves a crowd. It is also a great opportunity to sneak in some extra fertility boosting ingredients. In this case, you will be including collagen peptide powder in the pudding. Collagen is a supplement that is good for your reproductive health as well as your skin and bones.

Time: 15 minutes

Serving Size: 8

Prep Time: 15 minutes

Cook Time: 0 minutes

Nutritional Facts/Info: 236 calories, 7 g fat, 7 g protein, 37 g carbohydrates, 30 g sugar

Ingredients:

- 1 packet of banana pudding powder
- 2 cups whole milk (or per package directions)
- 1 can sweetened condensed milk (or per package directions)
- 3 bananas
- 1 cup whipped topping
- 1 scoop collagen peptide powder

Directions:

1. In a bowl combine the pudding powder, collagen peptide powder, and milks, whisk until thick and creamy. It may take a few minutes for the ingredients to fully combine.
2. Peel and slice the bananas into ½ inch slices.

3. In a casserole dish, layer pudding, bananas, and whipped topping in repeating layers until you've used all of the ingredients. Make the top layer the whipped topping.
4. Place in the fridge to chill until you are ready to serve.

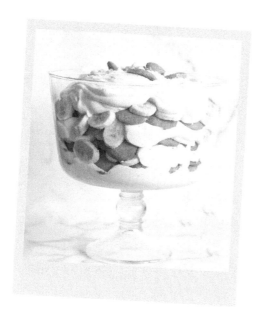

Chocolate Bark

This chocolate bark is packed with fertility superfoods! The chickpeas, cinnamon, and walnuts will boost fertility, all while satisfying any chocolate lover. Chocolate bark is relatively quick and easy to make, so long as you can be patient for three hours while it firms and cools in the fridge. It is easy to master this recipe and then tweak it for your personal favorite ingredients, like using a different kind of fertility friendly nut or including other plant-based proteins like sunflower seeds!

Time: 4 hours

Serving Size: 8

Prep Time: 20 minutes

Cook Time: 3 hours and 40 minutes

Nutritional Facts/Info:

341 calories, 19 g fat, 9 g protein, 37 g carbohydrates, 19 g sugar

Ingredients:

- 1 can chickpeas
- 1 tbsp coconut oil
- 1 tbsp cinnamon
- ¼ tsp salt
- 2 tbsp melted butter
- 1 cup semi-sweet chocolate chips
- ½ cup walnuts

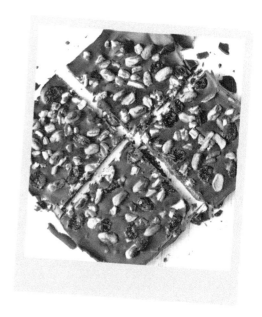

1. Preheat the oven to 400 °F.
2. Open the can of chickpeas and pour them into a strainer. Rinse well with cold water and pat dry.
3. Bake the chickpeas for eight to ten minutes, but check on them regularly as bake times can vary.
4. Remove from the oven and add the chickpeas to a bowl. Mix them with coconut oil, cinnamon, and salt. Then, place them back on the baking sheet and return to the oven.
5. Bake for 30 minutes.
6. Remove them from the heat and allow to cool to room temperature.
7. In a measuring cup, place 2 tbsp of butter and melt in the microwave. Once melted, measure out the chocolate chips, add to the butter, and microwave for roughly 30 seconds. Mix once heated and return to the microwave, melting slowly while stirring.
8. Combine the chickpeas, walnuts, and the melted chocolate in a bowl. Stir to fully combine.
9. Pour the chocolate chickpeas onto a baking sheet and spread the mixture until it is a thin sheet.
10. Place the dish in the refrigerator for at least 3 hours. Once firm, remove the chocolate bark from the fridge and break it apart into chunks and smaller pieces. Enjoy right away or store for several days!

Sweet Protein Bites

This no bake dessert is a great source of protein and sweetness. How many you make will depend on the size of the ball you create. Serving a crowd? It is simple to make smaller bites and feed the whole party. Serving just you and your spouse? Then feel free to make larger, indulgent bites.

Time: 10 minutes

Serving Size: Varies

Prep Time: 10 minutes

Cook Time: 0 minutes

Nutritional Facts/Info:

469 calories, 35 g fat, 16 g protein, 30 g carbohydrates, 11 g sugar

Ingredients:

- 1 cup rolled oats
- 1 cup shredded coconut
- 1 cup peanut butter
- ½ cup mini chocolate chips
- 1 tbsp cinnamon

Directions:

1. Add all of the ingredients to a large mixing bowl and stir until it forms a thick, loose shape.
2. Using your hands, roll small sections of the mixture into balls. You can decide how large or small to make these depending on how many servings you need.

3. Arrange the bites on a tray or tupperware and place in the fridge to cool and set before eating, this should not take more than 15 minutes.

4. Enjoy!

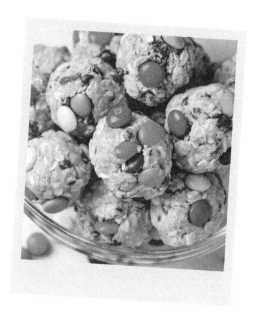

Berry Yogurt Bark

If chocolate isn't your sweet treat of choice, this recipe is a great way to enjoy a hand-held dessert, packed with fertility boosting ingredients, but avoiding chocolate. Once again, you'll need to be patient while it sets in the fridge or freezer, but the wait is worth it. If you are concerned about smashing the blueberries, then try this recipe with frozen berries! They will hold up better against the mixing process, but make sure to set them out for a few minutes before you begin.

Time: 3 hours and 10 minutes
Serving Size: 8
Prep Time: 3 hours and 10 minutes
Cook Time: 0 minutes
Nutritional Facts/Info: 126 calories, 6 g fat, 4 g protein, 15 g carbohydrates, 13 g sugar

Ingredients:

- 2 cups whole-fat vanilla yogurt
- ½ cup sunflower seeds
- ½ cup pomegranate seeds
- ½ cup blueberries
- ½ cup almonds
- ¼ cup honey

Directions:

1. In a large mixing bowl, combine all of the ingredients and mix (gently) until thoroughly combined. Mixing too vigorously can break the blueberries.

2. Spread the mixture out on a lined baking tray until it is roughly ½ inch thick across the sheet.
3. Place the baking tray in the fridge for roughly three hours while the bark firms.
4. Once firm, remove the bark from the fridge and break or snap into chunks.
5. Enjoy immediately or store in the fridge for several days.

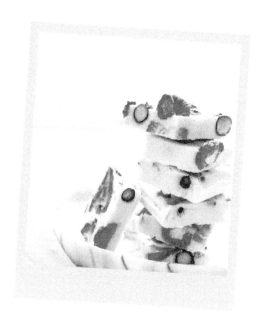

Fertility Cookies

How many fertility superfoods can you pack into one cookie? A lot! These cookies are delicious and nutritious. Best of all, they are great to serve as a dessert to friends and family, so your fertility diet doesn't need to go on pause just because you are serving a crowd. These are completely customizable so pick and choose the ingredients you like, and those you'd rather skip.

Time: 20 minutes

Serving Size: 36 cookies

Prep Time: 10 minutes

Cook Time: 10 minutes

Nutritional Facts/Info:

416 calories, 25 g fat, 9 g protein, 42 g carbohydrates, 13 g sugar

Ingredients:

- 3 cups rolled oats
- 1 cup butter
- 1 ½ cups flour
- 1 cup brown sugar
- 2 eggs
- 1 tsp baking soda
- 1 tsp salt
- 1 tbsp cinnamon
- 1 scoop collagen peptide powder
- ½ cup walnuts
- ½ cup dried cranberries
- ½ cup coconut flakes
- ¼ cup pumpkin seeds
- 2 tbsp chia seeds

Directions:

1. Preheat the oven to 350 °F.
2. In the large bowl of a stand mixer, combine sugar, butter, and eggs. Beat these until they form a smooth, thick consistency.
3. In a separate bowl, combine the flour, oats, baking soda, salt, cinnamon and collagen peptide powder.
4. Slowly add the dry ingredients into the wet while mixing on a low speed.
5. Once combined, add the cranberries, coconut, pumpkin seeds, walnuts, and chia seeds to the batter. It should become thick and clumpy.
6. Scoop one-inch balls of batter onto a lined baking sheet. They should be spaced roughly two inches apart, so you'll need to bake the cookies in batches.
7. Bake for 10 minutes.
8. Remove from the oven and allow to cool completely before enjoying.

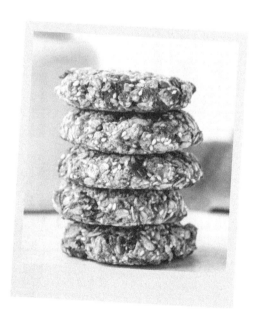

Avocado Chocolate Cake

Avocados are a commonly added ingredient to chocolate based desserts to add a healthy edge to a sweet treat. They are conveniently great for fertility! If you have a birthday or special evening approaching, look no further for a celebratory dish than this chocolate cake. If you love it like I do, it could even turn into your future baby's first birthday cake, taking your fertility diet full circle.

Time: 90 minutes

Serving Size: 8

Prep Time: 60 minutes

Cook Time: 30 minutes

Nutritional Facts/Info:

688 calories, 23 g fat, 8 g protein, 119 g carbohydrates, 73 g sugar

Cake Ingredients:

- 3 cups flour
- 5 tbsp cocoa powder
- 2 tsp baking powder
- 2 tsp baking soda
- 1 avocado
- ½ tsp salt
- ¼ cup vegetable oil
- 2 cups water
- 2 cups white vinegar
- 1 cup sugar
- ½ cup honey

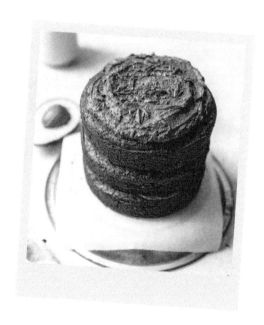

- 2 avocados
- 2 cups powdered sugar
- 4 tbsp cocoa powder

Directions:

1. Preheat the oven to 350 °F and line two round cake pans with parchment paper.
2. In a bowl, combine flour, cocoa powder, baking powder, baking soda, and salt.
3. Using a cutting board and a sharp knife, peel the avocado and remove the pit.
4. In a separate bowl, combine the avocado, oil, water, and vinegar. Whisk these ingredients until thoroughly combined. Then, pour them into the dry ingredients and stir.
5. When the mixture is halfway combined, add the sugar and honey to the bowl. Continue to mix until it is one homogenous batter.
6. Pour equal amounts of the batter into each cake pan.
7. Bake for 30 minutes.
8. While the cakes are baking, cut and peel two more avocados for the frosting. Mash these in a bowl.
9. Add the sugar and cocoa powder to the mashed avocados and beat with an electric mixer until the frosting forms stiff peaks. It should take about 5 minutes.
10. Set the frosting aside until the cakes are out of the oven and cooled.
11. Once they are finished baking, remove the cakes from the oven and allow them to cool for 30 minutes, removing them from their pans after 15.
12. To frost and assemble, place the first cake on a platter and add frosting to the top. Smooth the frosting with a rubber spatula. Place the second cake on top of the first and scoop frosting onto the top, smoothing in the same way. Then, add a generous amount of frosting to the sides of the cake. It is easiest to spin the plate or platter as you go, for a nice even spread of the frosting.
13. Enjoy!

Sweet Potato Bread

This sweet bread recipe is an alternative to banana or zucchini bread that relies on the fertility-friendly sweet potato for its sweetness, along with tasty spices and maple syrup. You can make this recipe with any variety of gluten free flour as well if you'd like to cut down on the traditional carbohydrates in baked goods. Be sure to do your research to see if the gluten free flour of your choice is a one to one replacement for traditional flour.

Time: 1 hour and 40 minutes

Serving Size: 6

Prep Time: 10 minutes

Cook Time: 90 minutes

Nutritional Facts/Info:

447 calories, 18 g fat, 7 g protein, 67 g carbohydrates, 23 g sugar

Ingredients:

- ¼ cup sugar
- ¼ cup brown sugar
- ¼ cup maple syrup
- ½ cup melted butter
- 2 eggs
- 1 ¾ cup flour
- cup milk
- 2 sweet potatoes
- 1 tsp baking soda
- ½ tsp salt
- 1 tbsp cinnamon
- ½ tsp nutmeg

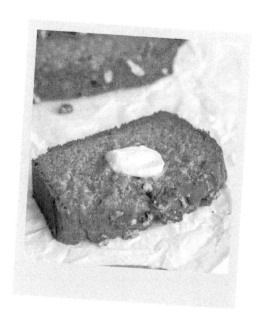

1. Preheat the oven to 350 °F.
2. Place the two sweet potatoes on a baking tray, poke the potatoes with a fork in a few spots, wrap in tinfoil, and bake for 30 minutes.
3. While the sweet potatoes bake, combine sugar, brown sugar, maple syrup and melted butter in a bowl until it forms a wet sand consistency.
4. Add both eggs to the sugar mixture and whisk vigorously until all the ingredients are combined.
5. In another bowl, combine the flour, baking soda, salt, and other seasonings.
6. Pour the dry ingredients slowly into the wet ingredients and stir until nearly combined.
7. When the sweet potatoes are done cooking, remove them from the oven. Allow to cool for a few minutes before peeling the skins and adding the peeled sweet potatoes to a bowl. Mash the sweet potatoes with a fork or potato masher. Once they are a smooth mixture, add them to the bowl with the remaining ingredients. Fold together.
8. Pour the batter into a greased bread pan and bake at 350 °F for one hour.
9. Remove from the oven and serve warm.

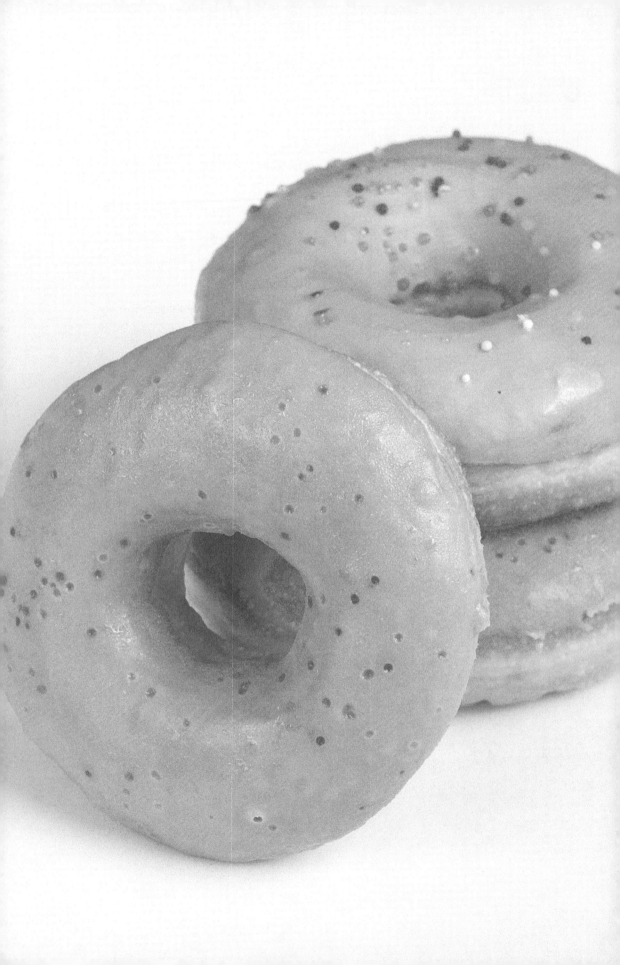

CHAPTER SEVEN

Snacks & Sides

No meal is complete without the perfect side dish or appetizer to compliment it. And, no afternoon is complete without the inevitable need for a midday snack. No worries, this book has you covered in both scenarios. Eating snacks or preparing sides for dinner still counts as far as your diet is concerned, so don't sway from the fertility boosting foods just because you're "only having a few." Taste test a few of my favorites like the chips and dip, oysters rockefeller dip, and the chickpea trail mix. Whether you like your snacks salty or sweet, there are endless options here. And, all of these dishes are rich in nutrients like protein, Vitamin A, and folic acid, which balance hormones, improve reproductive health, and strengthen reproductive material.

For best results, you'll want to make sure you have all the right tools in the kitchen. The most common tools required in these recipes are baking trays, pots and pans, and serving trays or dishes.

Pumpkin Hummus

Hummus is a great way for men and women to boost their fertility through healthy lentils and keep eating one of their favorite tasty snacks. There's no better way to enjoy a party platter of hummus than with close friends, so invite your fellow soon-to-be parents over for a bite and enjoy the healthy benefits!

Time: 50 minutes

Serving Size: 6

Prep Time: 10 minutes

Cook Time: 40 minutes

Nutritional Facts/Info: 434 calories, 36 g fat, 9 g protein, 24 g carbohydrates, 4 g sugar

Ingredients:

- 1 pumpkin
- 1 can garbanzo beans
- ¾ cup olive oil
- ¼ cup tahini
- 2 tbsp lemon juice
- 2 tsp minced garlic
- 1 tsp salt
- pepper and chili powder

Directions:

1. Preheat the oven to 425 °F.
2. Slice the pumpkin into wedges and remove the seeds. Arrange the slices on a baking tray and drizzle with olive oil.

3. Bake pumpkin for 40 minutes, flipping halfway.

4. Allow the pumpkin to cool for five to ten minutes after baking.

5. Once cooled, add the pumpkin slices to a food processor. Puree until smooth.

6. Add the garbanzo beans, tahini, lemon juice, minced garlic, and seasonings to the food processor. Pulse the mixture until mostly combined.

7. Slowly pour in the olive oil, continuing to pulse, until fully combined.

8. Taste and add additional seasonings depending on your taste preferences. If you like extra creamy hummus, add additional olive oil.

9. This dip is best served with veggies or crackers.

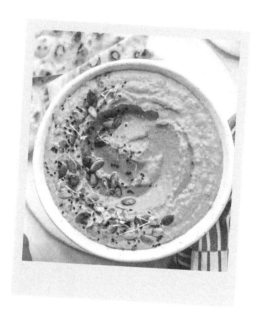

Crispy Asparagus

These crispy asparagus are an addicting treat that is also great for fertility. Asparagus contains folate, beneficial for both male and female fertility rates. And, they can be paired well with any main course. See the salmon recipe from Chapter 6 for a great pair.

Time: 25 minutes

Serving Size: 2 servings

Prep Time: 5 minutes

Cook Time: 20 minutes

Nutritional Facts/Info: 201 calories, 18 g fat, 4 g protein, 10 g carbohydrates, 3 g sugar

Ingredients:

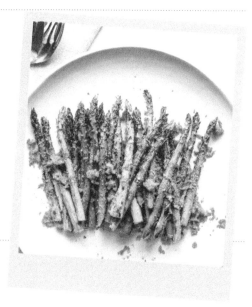

- 1 bunch of asparagus
- 2 tbsp minced garlic
- 3 tbsp melted butter
- 1 tsp onion powder
- 1 tsp salt
- 1 tsp pepper

Directions:

1. Preheat the oven to 400 °F.
2. Wash the bunch of asparagus.
3. Use a paring knife to whittle down the stems of the asparagus so they aren't as tough.
4. Spread the asparagus on a baking sheet and douse in melted butter.
5. Season with salt, pepper, minced garlic, and onion powder.
6. Bake for 20 minutes or until crispy.
7. Serve hot!

Roasted Sunflower Seeds

Sunflower seeds are great fertility boosters, especially for men. They are rich in vitamin E, zinc, and folic acid. Roasting sunflower seeds with your favorite seasonings makes a tasty and healthy snack. It is also a great snacking dish to serve at parties, little will your guests know all the health benefits they are eating.

Time: 35 minutes

Serving Size: 5 servings

Prep Time: 5 minutes

Cook Time: 30 minutes

Nutritional Facts/Info: 256 calories, 25 g fat, 6 g protein, 6 g carbohydrates, 1 g sugar

Ingredients:

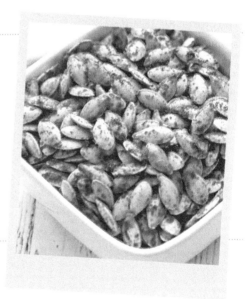

- 1 cup sunflower seeds
- ¼ cup olive oil
- 2 tsp salt
- 1 tsp paprika
- ½ tsp pepper

Directions:

1. Preheat the oven to 400 °F.
2. Line a baking sheet with parchment paper.
3. Combine the seasonings in a measuring cup.
4. Spread the sunflower seeds on the baking sheet and drizzle with olive oil and seasoning mix.
5. Bake for 30 minutes, flipping halfway.
6. Remove from the oven and allow to cool completely before snacking!

Chickpea Trail Mix

Homemade trail mix is always better than store bought alternatives, both because it tastes fresher and because you have control over what goes into the mix. When it comes to a trail mix that will improve the fertility health of women and men, there are a few superfoods that you can't miss. Like the namesake of this trail mix recipe, chickpeas! Make this trail mix for a movie-night with your partner or prepare ahead of time to use in your lunches all week.

Time: 60 minutes

Serving Size: 8

Prep Time: 10 minutes

Cook Time: 50 minutes

Nutritional Facts/Info:

313 calories, 15 g fat, 13 g protein, 35 g carbohydrates, 7 g sugar

Ingredients:

- 2 cups chickpeas
- ½ cup sunflower seeds
- ½ cup walnuts
- 1 cup cranberries
- 1 tbsp salt
- 2 tbsp garlic powder
- 1 tsp smoked paprika
- ¼ cup melted butter

1. Preheat the oven to 250 °F.
2. In a bowl, combine chickpeas, sunflower seeds, and walnuts. Dust with seasonings and melted butter.
3. Stir the dry ingredients until thoroughly coated.
4. Spread the ingredients across a baking sheet.
5. Bake for 50 minutes, stirring on the pan every fifteen minutes.
6. Once thoroughly roasted, remove from the oven and allow to cool.
7. In a bowl, combine the dried cranberries with the toasted ingredients. Toss to combine.
8. Enjoy right away or store in air-tight containers to enjoy throughout the week.

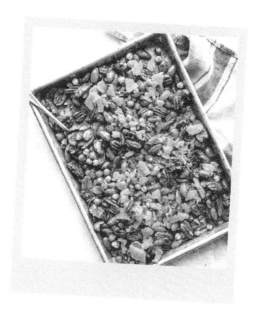

Brazil Nut Mix

Brazil nuts contain the antioxidant known as selenium. Selenium improves the health of ovarian follicles, essential in the process of releasing a healthy egg. The best sources of selenium can be found in Brazil nuts where just a single nut contains all the selenium you need in your daily diet. Of course, these nuts are so tasty you won't want to stop at just one.

Time: 35 minutes
Serving Size: 5
Prep Time: 5 minutes
Cook Time: 30 minutes
Nutritional Facts/Info:
706 calories, 55 g fat, 14 g protein, 48 g carbohydrates, 6 g sugar

Ingredients:

- 1 ½ cups Brazil nuts
- 2 cups gluten-free chex cereal
- ½ cup almonds
- ½ cup gluten free pretzels
- ¼ cup dried cranberries
- 2 tsp salt
- 1 tbsp garlic powder
- ¼ cup melted butter

Directions:

1. Preheat the oven to 400 °F.
2. Add the nuts, cereal, and dried fruit to a bowl. Drizzle melted butter over the ingredients and mix thoroughly. Then, dust with the seasonings and mix again.

3. Cover a baking sheet with parchment paper.

4. Spread the mix across the baking sheet making sure there isn't much overlap.

5. Bake for 30 minutes, flipping every ten minutes.

6. Remove from the heat and cool to room temperature.

7. Enjoy! This trail mix can be stored in tupperware and enjoyed for several days after baking.

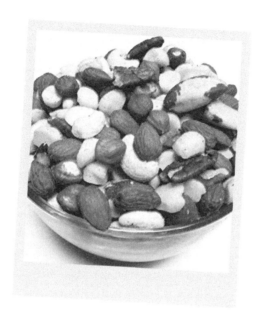

Spinach Balls

As we've established, spinach is a leafy green vegetable that is great for fertility. But inventive spinach based recipes don't stop with salads! Spinach balls can be eaten as a snack or served as a side to your favorite dinners and lunches. They are nutrient rich treats that pack in the vegetables without you even realizing it.

Time: 35 minutes

Serving Size: 10

Prep Time: 10 minutes

Cook Time: 25 minutes

Nutritional Facts/Info: 219 calories, 16 g fat, 11 g protein, 10 g carbohydrates, 1 g sugar

Ingredients:

- 1 box frozen spinach
- 3 tbsp garlic
- ½ cup Parmesan cheese
- ½ cup softened butter
- 2 eggs
- 1 cup bread crumbs
- Salt and pepper

Directions:

1. Prior to cooking, take the frozen spinach out of the freezer and allow it to partially thaw.
2. Preheat the oven to 350 °F.

3. Once thawed, combine spinach, garlic, butter, cheese, eggs, bread crumbs, and seasonings in a bowl. The consistency should resemble a cookie dough once mixed.
4. Scoop out tablespoon sized balls of the mixture, roll between your palms until smooth and arrange on a baking tray.
5. Cook the spinach balls for 25 minutes.
6. Remove from the oven and allow the spinach balls to cool for five minutes before serving.

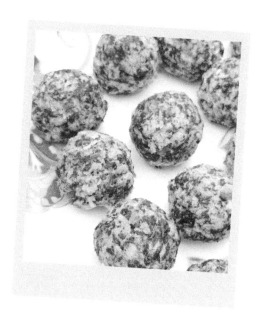

Fertility Charcuterie Boards

Charcuterie boards have gained lots of popularity in recent years. They are fun to serve at parties and family dinners, at date nights or even girls nights. You can pick and choose your favorite ingredients to add to a charcuterie board, including fertility friendly ingredients. These are my favorite ingredients that boost fertility and make for a fun charcuterie board. For this board in particular, you can order beef liver jerky from online or you can make the jerky yourself.

Time: 27 minutes
Serving Size: 8
Prep Time: 15 minutes
Cook Time: 12 minutes
Nutritional Facts/Info:
342 calories, 26 g fat, 19 g protein, 10 g carbohydrates, 3 g sugar

Ingredients:

- ¼ cup sunflower seeds
- ½ cup walnuts
- 1 cup beef liver jerky
- 1 cup sliced cheese of your choice
- 15 almond nut thin crackers
- 4 eggs
- 3 tbsp mustard
- 3 tbsp whole-fat plain yogurt
- 1 tsp paprika
- 1 avocado

1. Place a pot of water to boil on the stove.
2. Once boiling, add the whole eggs to the water and immediately cut the heat. Allow the eggs to sit in the water for 8 minutes.
3. While the eggs cook, slice the avocado in half. Remove the skins and the pit, then slice the avocado into thin slices.
4. Remove the hard boiled eggs from the water and immediately rinse in cold water. Peel away the egg shell and place the eggs onto a cutting board.
5. Cut each egg in half and spoon out the yolk into a bowl.
6. Stir the yolks with the yogurt and mustard until the mixture is thoroughly combined. Spoon that mixture back into the wells of the egg whites. Sprinkle them with paprika.
7. To arrange the charcuterie board, pick your favorite serving platter and place the jerky, crackers, cheese slices, avocado slices, and deviled eggs around the board. Pour the walnuts and sunflower seeds into small bowls and place those on the platter.
8. Enjoy!

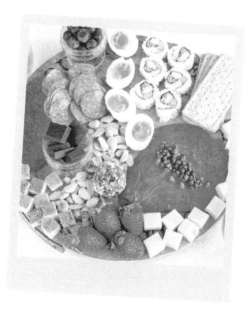

Chips and Dip

Just because you are following a fertility diet, doesn't mean you need to give up indulgent snacks like chips and dip. Making a homemade guac is a great way to pack in fertility boosting foods like avocados. And, avoid the extra carbs by choosing a nut-based cracker.

Time: 10 minutes

Serving Size: 4

Prep Time: 10 minutes

Cook Time: 0 minutes

Nutritional Facts/Info: 460 calories, 23 g fat, 8 g protein, 57 g carbohydrates, 1 g sugar

Ingredients:

- 2 avocados
- 1 lime
- ¼ cup cilantro
- ½ red onion
- 1 package almond based nut thins

Directions:

1. Slice each of the avocados in half. Peel the skins and remove the pits.
2. Chop the red onion into small pieces. You will only need half the onion, reserve the rest for a later snack.
3. Pick the leaves from the stems of the cilantro. Slice them into smaller sections.
4. Chop one lime in half and set aside.
5. Add the meat of the avocado to a bowl and mash with a fork until smooth.

6. Add the cilantro and red onions to the bowl, mix to combine. Once combined, squirt with lime juice and stir lightly.

7. Serve with a platter of nut thins and enjoy!

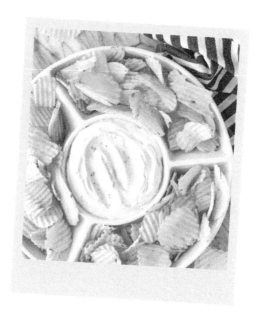

Sunflower Seed Crisps

Sunflower seeds can be hard to eat in large quantities, but this recipe solves that problem. Eat all the fertility-boosting sunflower seeds you want from these sweet and savory sunflower seed crisps. They don't need to spend any time in the oven! And, they make great snacks as well as sides for your favorite lunches and entrees.

Time: 15 minutes

Serving Size: 10

Prep Time: 5 minutes

Cook Time: 10 minutes

Nutritional Facts/Info: 202 calories, 8 g fat, 2 g protein, 32 g carbohydrates, 30 g sugar

Ingredients:

- 2 cups sunflower seeds
- 1 cup sugar
- ½ cup water
- ½ cup maple syrup
- 2 tbsp butter
- 1 tsp salt
- ½ tsp baking soda
- 1 tbsp vegetable oil

Directions:

1. Place a saucepan on the stove over medium heat.
2. Line a baking sheet with parchment paper and drizzle the paper with roughly 1 tbsp of oil to avoid sticking later.

3. Combine the sugar, water, and maple syrup in the pan. Stir the ingredients together and bring to a boil. The newly forming carmel should turn a light brown.

4. Remove the pot from the heat and quickly stir in the butter, salt, and baking soda.

5. Before the mixture sets, add the sunflower seeds. Stir until thick and sticky.

6. Spread the mixture out onto the prepared baking sheet. It will harden quickly, so be sure to work fast. It should be an even width all the way across the sheet.

7. Once fully cooled, break into pieces.

8. Enjoy immediately or save for sweet and savory treats throughout the week.

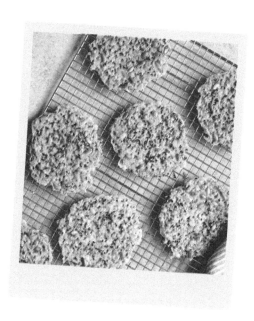

Fried Sardines

Sardines are one of those fertility friendly foods that are more difficult to incorporate into your everyday diet, but by breading and frying these fertility boosting fish, you can easily eat them as a snack or appetizer.

Time: 35 minutes

Serving Size: 6

Prep Time: 20 minutes

Cook Time: 15 minutes

Nutritional Facts/Info:

390 calories, 26 g fat, 17 g protein, 21 g carbohydrates, 1 g sugar

Ingredients:

- 12 sardines
- ½ cup flour
- 2 eggs
- 1 cup bread crumbs
- ½ cup vegetable oil
- Salt and pepper

Directions:

1. Rinse the sardines under cool water and towel them dry.
2. Arrange one bowl of whisked eggs and one bowl of bread crumbs. You can place the flour in a bowl or plastic bag, whatever breading method works better for you will work for this recipe.

3. Once the breading station is prepared, place two or three sardines at a time in the flour and shake or stir until coated. Move the sardines from the flour to the egg wash. Turn them with a fork until thoroughly covered in egg. Finally, add the damp sardines to the bread crumb bowls and cover them heavily in bread crumbs. Repeat for all 12 sardines.
4. Pour the oil into a high-sided frying pan and place on the stove over high heat.
5. To check the oil temperature, flick water into the pan. If the oil sizzles at the touch of water, it is ready.
6. Using a pair of tongs, place four sardines at a time in the oil. Fry them for two minutes on each side, turning as needed. They should turn golden brown.
7. Remove the sardines from the oil and place on a wire rack to cool. Be careful not to crowd the pan, as that can lower the oil temperature drastically.
8. Continue the process until all the sardines are fried.
9. Serve warm and enjoy!

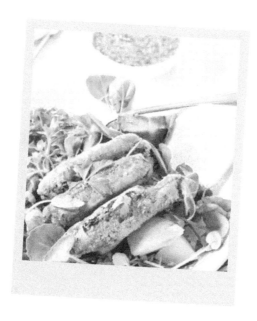

Asparagus Casserole

Asparagus casserole is a creative spin off green bean casserole. It is a great holiday replacement dish to lean into the fertility diet, or a fantastic side to make anytime of year! It feeds a crowd, so come hungry!

Time: 65 minutes

Serving Size: 8

Prep Time: 15 minutes

Cook Time: 50 minutes

Nutritional Facts/Info: 188 calories, 12 g fat, 7 g protein, 15 g carbohydrates, 6 g sugar

Ingredients:

- 2 ½ lb asparagus
- 4 tbsp butter
- 1 cup mushrooms
- ½ white onion
- ¼ cup flour
- 1 ¼ cup milk
- ¼ cup mayo
- ½ cup whole-fat plain yogurt
- 1 cup mozzarella cheese
- 1 tsp salt
- 1 tsp paprika
- 6 oz fried onion topping

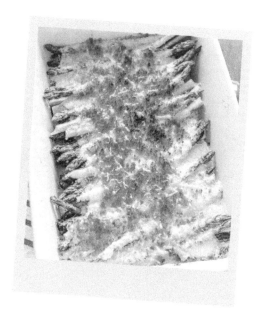

1. Preheat the oven to 350 °F.
2. Using a knife and cutting board, mince the onion into small pieces. You will only need half of the onion. Chop the mushrooms into halves or quarters per your preference.
3. Place a pan on the stove to medium heat. Add the butter to the pan and wait for it to melt. Once melted, add the onion, mushrooms, and asparagus to the pan. Cook for five to eight minutes.
4. Pour the flour over the cooking vegetables and cook for an additional two minutes.
5. Turn the heat to low and slowly pour the milk into the vegetable mixture. The heat should stay low to prevent the milk from turning grainy.
6. Once the mixture is thick, add the mayonnaise, yogurt, cheese, and seasonings to the pot.
7. Remove from heat and stir in   of the can of fried onion topping.
8. Pour the entire mixture into a greased baking sheet. Arrange the mixture until it is level all the way across.
9. Top with the remaining fried onions.
10. Bake for 30 minutes.
11. When finished baking, remove the casserole from the oven and allow it to set for five minutes.
12. Serve as a side to your favorite dinner and enjoy!

Granola Bars

Granola bars are the perfect on the go snack, but those bought from the grocery store are often full of unwanted ingredients and chemicals. Lucky for fertility dieters, making your own granola bars is easy! And, this recipe is packed with fertility friendly ingredients that will balance your hormones while you snack.

Time: 1 hour and 10 minutes

Serving Size: 8

Prep Time: 1 hour and 10 minutes

Cook Time: 0 minutes

Nutritional Facts/Info:

406 calories, 21 g fat, 13 g protein, 47 g carbohydrates, 25 g sugar

Ingredients:

- 1 cup crunchy peanut butter
- ½ cup honey
- 1 tsp vanilla
- 2 ½ cups oats
- ½ cup sunflower seeds
- ¼ cup dried cranberries
- 1 tsp salt
- ½ cup dark chocolate chips

Directions:

1. Scoop the peanut butter into a microwave safe bowl and microwave for 20 to 30 seconds or until it is easy to stir.
2. Add the maple syrup and vanilla to the softened peanut butter and stir to combine.

3. In a separate bowl, measure out the oats, sunflower seeds, and dried cranberries. Slowly pour the dry ingredients into the peanut butter mixture, stirring as you go.

4. Once the ingredients are evenly combined, add the chocolate chips to the bowl and stir again.

5. Line a 9 x 13 baking pan with parchment paper, add a bit of water to the pan first if you are having trouble getting the paper to lay flat.

6. Pour the granola bar mixture into the pan and flatten with a spatula until the mixture is level.

7. Place in the fridge for one hour or overnight. Once set, cut into slices and serve or save for snacks all week!

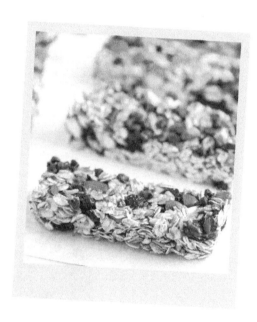

Veggie Medley

Want a vegetable side dish with your fertility diet dinner but not sure which veggie to whip up? Or, wanting a bowl of veggies without eating salad? How about all of them? This side dish will perfectly compliment any dinner, and it is packed with fertility friendly vegetables.

Time: 50 minutes

Serving Size: 4

Prep Time: 15 minutes

Cook Time: 35 minutes

Nutritional Facts/Info: 385 calories, 38 g fat, 5 g protein, 12 g carbohydrates, 3 g sugar

Ingredients:

- 1 cup asparagus
- 2 cups spinach
- 1 head cauliflower
- 1 cup brussel sprouts
- ¾ cup olive oil
- ¼ cup soy sauce
- 3 tbsp garlic
- 2 tsp salt
- 1 tbsp chili powder
- 1 tsp red pepper flakes

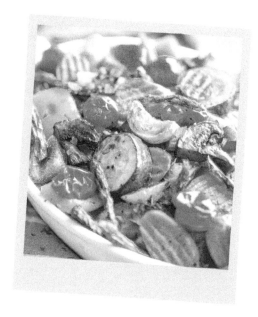

1. Preheat the oven to 375 °F.
2. Rinse all of the veggies in cold water and pat them dry with a paper or cloth towel.
3. Using a cutting board and sharp knife, slice the butts of the brussel sprouts away from the bulb of the vegetable. Then, cut the brussel sprouts into fourths. Collect all the pieces and leaves into a bowl. Cut the cauliflower florets away from the main stem to a size of your choosing. You can chop them as small as you like. Add the cauliflower to the bowl with the brussel sprouts.
4. Season the cauliflower and brussel sprouts with ¼ cup of the olive oil, half the salt, 1 tbsp of garlic powder, and the chili powder. Stir until the seasonings thoroughly coat all of the vegetables.
5. Spread the vegetables on a baking sheet and bake for 25 minutes.
6. While the brussel sprouts and cauliflower cook, chop off the thick ends of the asparagus.
7. When there is only a few minutes of cooking time left for the vegetables in the oven, add a wok or pan to the stove top on medium heat. Drizzle with a splash of olive oil.
8. Once hot, add the asparagus and spinach to the pan. Stir continuously and season with the remaining garlic powder, salt, and olive oil. These should cook for about five minutes before the other vegetables are added.
9. When the brussel sprouts and cauliflower are done cooking, remove them from the oven and immediately toss into the pan with the other vegetables.
10. Season the entire mixture with soy sauce and red pepper flakes and cook for an additional five minutes.
11. Remove the vegetables from the heat and serve while hot.
12. Enjoy!

Quinoa Dinner Side

This quinoa dinner side dish is a great addition to any weekend cookouts or meaty main courses. It packs in the fertility friendly vegetables and proteins with a fresh taste. You can cook the quinoa per the package directions, and I advise making more than a single cup so that there is enough base for the other vegetables to mix in.

Time: 20 minutes

Serving Size: 2

Prep Time: 5 minutes

Cook Time: 15 minutes

Nutritional Facts/Info: 517 calories, 9 g fat, 23 g protein, 89 g carbohydrates, 6 g sugar

Ingredients:

- 1 package quinoa
- ½ cup chickpeas
- 1 head of broccoli
- 1 tsp salt
- 1 tsp paprika
- ½ tsp oregano
- 1 tbsp lemon juice

Directions:

1. Cook the quinoa per package directions.
2. Rinse the chickpeas in cool water and pat dry with a paper towel. Set these aside for later.

3. Rinse the broccoli in cool water. Then, using a cutting board and sharp knife, separate the florets from the stem. Cut these as small as you would like.

4. When the quinoa is half way cooked, add the broccoli to the pot with an extra splash of water and stir. Cover with a lid so the broccoli can steam for the remaining cook time of the quinoa.

5. When the quinoa has reached its total cook time, add the chickpeas and all of the seasonings to the pot. Stir the ingredients until they are evenly distributed. Allow the mixture to cook together for three minutes, or until the chickpeas are warm.

6. Serve immediately as a side to your favorite dinner.

7. Enjoy!

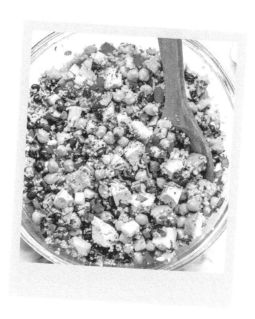

Italian Chickpea Bread

The general rule is that fertility diet followers should cut down on their simple sugars and carbohydrates. This can leave bread lovers feeling down. Never fear, this recipe is a homemade bread option for soon-to-be parents that makes a great side dish at dinner. It has a lovely Italian-based seasoning and relies on chickpea flour instead of traditional flour.

Time: 3 hours and 30 minutes

Serving Size: 6

Prep Time: 3 hours and 15 minutes

Cook Time: 15 minutes

Nutritional Facts/Info: 167 calories, 7 g fat, 6 g protein, 21 g carbohydrates, 4 g sugar

Ingredients:

- 1 cup chickpea flour
- 1 cup water
- 2 tbsp olive oil
- 2 tsp Italian seasoning
- 2 tsp rosemary
- 1 tsp salt
- ½ tsp black pepper

Directions:

1. Combine the flour and water in a bowl. Whisk the ingredients together until they are smooth and allow the mixture to set at room temperature for three hours.
2. Preheat the oven to 450 °F and grease a nine inch baking pan.

3. If a foam has formed on the top of the flour and water mixture, scoop it away. Add the olive oil and seasonings at this time, stirring them in lightly.
4. Pour the mixture into the pan and salt the top.
5. Bake for 15 minutes or until the crust is golden brown.
6. Remove the fully baked bread from the oven and allow it to cool for five minutes. Once cooled, slice into the bread.
7. Serve warm and enjoy!

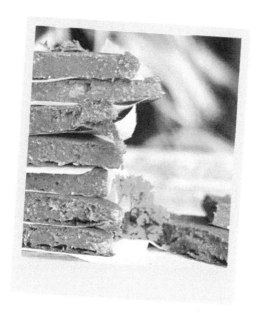

Macaroni Salad

Macaroni salads are the perfect side dish to serve at a summer cookout. They are cool and refreshing, with a serving of healthy vegetables. In this recipe, I've replaced standard pasta with chickpea pasta. Not only is this option gluten free for any soon-to-be parents who can't eat gluten, but it is made from the fertility boosting chickpeas that we love so much. Unlike most macaroni salads, this recipe uses asparagus, another fertility superfood, so you can serve a side that follows your diet perfectly!

Time: 30 minutes

Serving Size: 4

Prep Time: 20 minutes

Cook Time: 10 minutes

Nutritional Facts/Info:

713 calories, 21 g fat, 48 g protein, 104 g carbohydrates, 18 g sugar

Ingredients:

- 1 box chickpea pasta
- 2 cups chopped asparagus
- 1 stalk celery
- ¼ onion
- ¼ cup mayonnaise
- ½ cup cubed cheddar cheese
- 1 tsp onion powder
- 1 tsp salt

1. Cook the chickpea pasta per package instructions, once strained from the boiling water, immediately spray in cold water and set the cooked noodles in the fridge to cool for 15 minutes.
2. Using a cutting board and sharp knife, chop the asparagus into chunks. Finley mince ¼ of one onion and chop one stalk of celery.
3. Mix all the vegetables together with the mayonnaise, cheese cubes, and seasonings.
4. Once the noodles have cooled, add them to the bowl and stir until all the ingredients are evenly distributed.
5. Serve cool and enjoy!

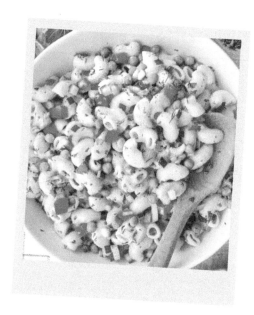

Oysters Rockefeller Dip

This addictive side dish will quickly become a family favorite. It is also an easy way to eat the fertility friendly oysters, hardly knowing they are in the dish! No need to shuck fresh oysters and turn your kitchen into an operating table, simply buy the canned variety. Serve this dip at family dinners or parties with your favorite crackers or breads, it is sure to be a hit!

Time: 35 minutes

Serving Size: 6

Prep Time: 10 minutes

Cook Time: 25 minutes

Nutrition Facts/Info: 226 calories, 14 g fat, 13 g protein, 13 g carbohydrates, 5 g sugar

Ingredients:

- 12 fresh oysters or 2 cans of oysters
- 1 cup whole-fat plain yogurt
- ½ cup mayonnaise
- 3 cups spinach
- 2 green onions
- ¼ cup Parmesan cheese
- 1 tbsp butter
- 1 tsp garlic powder
- 2 tsp Worcestershire sauce
- 1 tsp salt
- 1 tsp pepper

1. Preheat the oven to 350 °F.
2. Place a pan on the oven over medium heat and add butter to melt. Once melted, add the oysters to the pan and cook for one to two minutes or until just seared on the outside. Remove the pan from the heat.
3. In a bowl, combine the yogurt, mayonnaise, and lemon juice. Mix the ingredients thoroughly.
4. Using a cutting board and a sharp knife, chop the green onions into ½ inch pieces.
5. Add the spinach, green onions, Parmesan cheese, and seasonings to the yogurt mixture. Stir until all the ingredients are evenly distributed.
6. Slowly add the seared oysters to the bowl, you may chop any particularly large oysters in half or quarters. Stir all the ingredients together.
7. Pour the mixture into a casserole dish and bake for 25 minutes. The final consistency should resemble spinach and artichoke dip, thick but loose enough to dip into with a cracker.
8. Serve with your favorite dipping vehicles like crackers, toasts, or veggies, and enjoy!

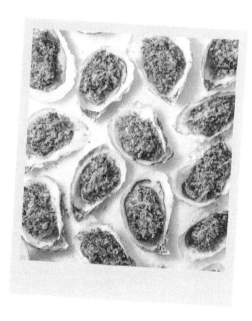

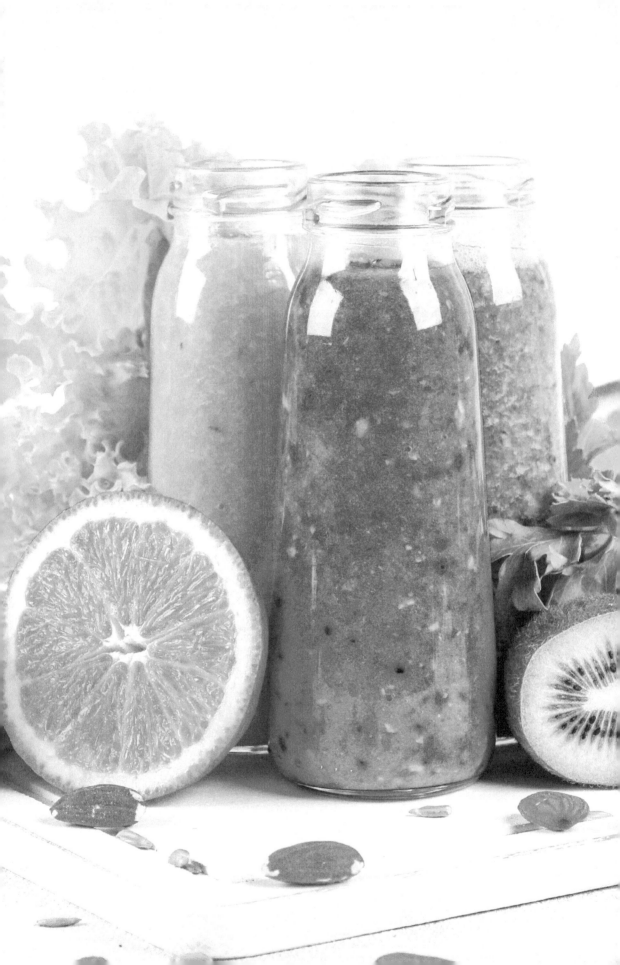

CHAPTER EIGHT

Drinks

Last but not least, don't forget to serve yourself a drink. Some of these options, like the smoothies, can serve as meal replacements or mid day snacks if you prefer to drink your nutrients. They are also perfect to enjoy after a run or workout class. Our other drink choices include mocktails and teas, so that even soon-to-be parents have a glass to carry around a party. Taste test my favorites like the peanut butter protein smoothie, hot chocolate, and citrus mocktail. The common ingredients in these drinks like collagen peptide powder, goji berries, and even avocado are rich in the vitamins and nutrients that soon-to-be parents rely on for a happy conception journey. Remember, be sure to ask your doctor before taking any supplements or adding dietary supplements to your meals. They will have information on how these compounds affect you specifically.

For best results, you'll want to make sure you have all the right tools in the kitchen. The most common tools required in these recipes include a blender, a cocktail shaker, and a tea kettle.

Peanut Butter Protein Smoothie

Adding peanut butter and spinach to smoothies is a great way to pack a smoothie with protein and the healthy nutrients you might miss out on throughout the day. Because fertility can be improved through whole-fat dairies, be sure to use whole milk and full fat yogurt in your smoothies. Always consult a doctor before adding any supplements, including collagen peptides, to your foods. This recipe will work just as well without the powder if it isn't best for your unique situation.

Time: 5 minutes
Serving Size: 1
Prep Time: 5 minutes
Cook Time: 0 minutes
Nutritional Facts/Info:
639 calories, 41 g fat, 27 g protein, 52 g carbohydrates, 33 g sugar

Ingredients:

- ¼ cup peanut butter
- 1 banana
- 1 cup spinach
- ½ cup full fat yogurt
- ½ cup whole milk
- 1 scoop collagen peptide powder

Directions:

1. Add all ingredients to a single serving blender.
2. Blend until smooth, adding more milk as necessary to find your favorite smoothie consistency.
3. Enjoy it cold!

Blueberry Ovulation Smoothie

This berry smoothie includes the vitamins that are essential during ovulation. For best results enjoy this smoothie on days 10 through 15 of your ovulation cycle. Estrogen levels spike during ovulation, so eating and drinking foods that can properly metabolize estrogen is essential.

Time: 5 minutes

Serving Size: 1

Prep Time: 5 minutes

Cook Time: 0 minutes

Nutritional Facts/Info:

341 calories, 16 g fat, 13 g protein, 44 g carbohydrates, 16 g sugar

Ingredients:

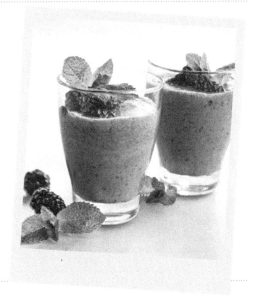

- ½ cup kale
- 1 cup mix of frozen blueberries and blackberries
- 1 tbsp sunflower seeds
- 1 tbsp flax seed
- 1 banana
- 1 tsp maca powder
- 2 cups whole milk

Directions:

1. Remove the stems from the kale before measuring the ½ cup.
2. Add all ingredients to a blender and blend until smooth, roughly 30 seconds.
3. Enjoy cold!

Chocolate Shake

Have a sweet tooth? This shake is the perfect blend of healthy and sweet that is jam packed with the ingredients you need to boost fertility. This is a great treat to make with your partner for a quick dessert. Want to make it even sweeter? Add whipped cream to your shake!

Time: 5 minutes

Serving Size: 1

Prep Time: 5 minutes

Cook Time: 0 minutes

Nutritional Facts/Info:

557 calories, 43 g fat, 8 g protein, 47 g carbohydrates, 20 g sugar

Ingredients:

- 1 banana
- ½ avocado
- ½ cup coconut milk
- 1 tbsp cocoa powder
- 1 tsp maca powder
- 1 tsp vanilla

Directions:

1. Begin by cutting the avocado in half, removing the pit, and peeling off the skin. Chop one half of the avocado into smaller chunks.
2. Peel and chop one banana into pieces as well. For an extra cold shake, freeze your banana and avocado chunks ahead of time.
3. Add all ingredients to a blender and blend until smooth, roughly 30 seconds.
4. Enjoy cold!

Citrus Smoothie

Citrus fruits are fertility superfoods, and they can make refreshing smoothies too. This smoothie relies on oranges, grapefruit, and lemon to pack in the citrus. Plus, I've added spinach so you get an extra serving of Vitamin A and other fertility boosting nutrients in your cup.

Time: 5 minutes

Serving Size: 1

Prep Time: 5 minutes

Cook Time: 0 minutes

Nutritional Facts/Info: 175 calories, 4 g fat, 6 g protein, 29 g carbohydrates, 24 g sugar

Ingredients:

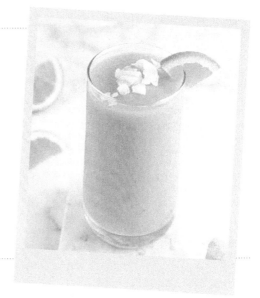

- ½ cup orange juice
- ½ cup whole-fat plain yogurt
- ½ cup spinach
- 1 scoop ice
- ½ cup sliced grapefruit
- 1 tbsp lemon juice

Directions:

1. Peel and slice a grapefruit. You will use roughly half the grapefruit. Reserve the remaining half of the grapefruit for a future smoothie.
2. Add the grapefruit to the blender with orange juice, yogurt, spinach, ice, and lemon juice.
3. Blend together for roughly one minute or until everything is icey and smooth.
4. Enjoy it cold!

Acai Smoothie

Acai is a great fruit for fertility, because it is a low glycemic fruit. Meaning, this fruit will not spike your blood sugar. It is commonly used in smoothie bowls, or acai bowls, so if you'd prefer to enjoy this smoothie in a bowl, go for it!

Time: 5 minutes

Serving Size: 1

Prep Time: 5 minutes

Cook Time: 0 minutes

Nutritional Facts/Info:

706 calories, 55 g fat, 23 g protein, 38 g carbohydrates, 16 g sugar

Ingredients:

- ½ cup frozen acai berries or smoothie mix
- 1 cup spinach
- ¼ cup almond butter
- 1 cup whole milk
- 2 tbsp chia seeds

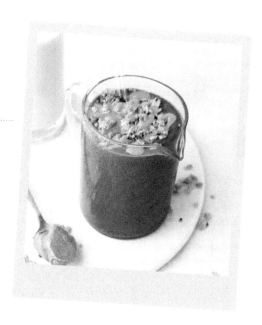

Directions:

1. Chop the stems from the spinach leaves.
2. Add all the ingredients to a blender and blend until smooth, roughly 30 seconds.
3. Enjoy cold!

Orange Goji Berry Smoothie

Goji berries are a fertility superfood. They have a low glycemic index, but they are packed with important vitamins and nutrients. While this fruit may sound exotic, you can find it at any local grocery store. Most of them are dried, so you'll need to soak the berries for 10 to 15 minutes prior to adding to any smoothies.

Time: 10 minutes

Serving Size: 1

Prep Time: 10 minutes

Cook Time: 0 minutes

Nutritional Facts/Info:

692 calories, 20 g fat, 26 g protein, 108 g carbohydrates, 67 g sugar

Ingredients:

- 1 cup whole milk
- 1 banana
- ¼ cup goji berries
- 1 tbsp almond butter
- 1 tbsp flaxseed
- ½ tsp cinnamon
- ½ tsp grated ginger

Directions:

1. Place the goji berries in a bowl of water to soak for ten minutes.
2. Once soaked, add the berries, milk banana, and all other ingredients to a blender.
3. Blend until smooth, roughly 45 seconds, and enjoy!

Hot Chocolate

You can still enjoy a cozy hot chocolate while focusing on your fertility diet. Including key protein powders with your cocoa powder is an easy way to slip extra nutrients into your diet while drinking a childhood favorite of your own.

Time: 8 minutes

Serving Size: 2

Prep Time: 3 minutes

Cook Time: 5 minutes

Nutritional Facts/Info:

657 calories, 27 g fat, 47 g protein, 69 g carbohydrates, 63 g sugar

Ingredients:

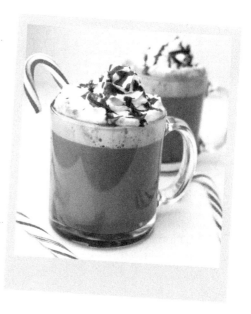

- 3 cups whole milk
- 2 tbsp sugar
- 4 tbsp cocoa powder
- 2 scoops collagen peptide powder

Directions:

1. Pour the milk into two mugs and stir in the sugar.
2. Microwave the milk and sugar mixtures for two minutes.
3. Next, stir in the cocoa powder and collagen peptide powder to the liquid. Microwave for an additional two minutes.
4. Continue to stir and microwave until all of the powder has been absorbed.
5. Enjoy hot and top with your favorite hot chocolate toppings like whipped cream or candy canes.

Citrus Mocktail

Citrus fruits are great fertility boosters, and during a time of your life when you can't indulge in an alcoholic drink, it is nice to enjoy something close. Citrus fruits are full of Vitamin C, folate, and calcium, making them a great option for anyone looking to boost their fertility. Serve this mocktail in a fun glass for an even brighter drinking experience.

Time: 3 minutes

Serving Size: 1

Prep Time: 3 minutes

Cook Time: 0 minutes

Nutritional Facts/Info: 51 calories, 0 g fat, 1 g protein, 11 g carbohydrates, 9 g sugar

Ingredients:

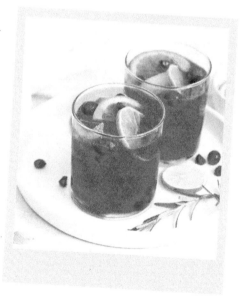

- 3 oz fresh squeezed orange juice
- 1 oz sparkling water
- 1 oz lemon juice
- Scoop of ice
- Lemon wedge

Directions:

1. Using a traditional shot measuring glass, measure out the orange juice, sparkling water, and lemon juice into a cocktail shaker.
2. Add a scoop of ice to the shaker and shake for 30 seconds.
3. Strain into a glass and add a few more ice cubes. Slice a wedge from your lemon to garnish the side of the glass and enjoy!

Virgin Mojito

Mojitos are another refreshing cocktail that can easily be transformed into a mocktail for soon-to-be mothers. The citrus juice and mint in these drinks are great for your fertility health.

Time: 5 minutes

Serving Size: 1

Prep Time: 5 minutes

Cook Time: 0 minutes

Nutritional Facts/Info: 77 calories, 0 g fat, 1 g protein, 22 g carbohydrates, 2 g sugar

Ingredients:

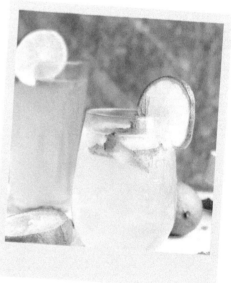

- 1 bunch of mint leaves
- 1 ounce lime juice
- ½ ounce simple syrup
- 4 ounces club soda
- Scoop of ice
- Lime wedge

Directions:

1. Add mint leaves, lime juice and simple syrup to a glass. Using a muddler, or end of a wooden spoon if you don't have an official muddler, muddle the mint leaves.
2. Pour the club soda into the glass.
3. Add ice and garnish with a wedge of lime on the edge of the glass.
4. Enjoy!

Virgin Margarita

No taco night is complete without a margarita, but when you are trying to start a family or are pregnant, a standard margarita is not what the doctor orders. This recipe will serve all the refreshing goodness of a regular margarita, and none of the disastrous effects. I've included strawberries in this recipe, but you can swap those out for another fruit of your choice or jalapenos if you prefer spice.

Time: 5 minutes
Serving Size: 1
Prep Time: 5 minutes
Cook Time: 0 minutes
Nutritional Info/Facts: 135 calories, 0 g fat, 1 g protein, 35 g carbohydrates, 7 g sugar

Ingredients:

- 3 oz club soda
- 2 oz orange juice
- 1 oz lime juice
- 3 strawberries
- 1 oz simple syrup
- Scoop of ice

Directions:

1. Rinse the strawberries in cool water. Cut off the stems and slice the strawberries into quarters.
2. Add a scoop of ice to a cocktail shaker.
3. Measure out and pour the orange juice, lime juice, and simple syrup into the shaker.

4. Add the strawberry slices to the shaker.
5. Shake vigorously for two minutes. You can use a towel to hold the shaker when it gets cold.
6. Strain into a glass until it is half full, top the rest of the way with club soda.
7. Garnish the glass with a strawberry and enjoy!

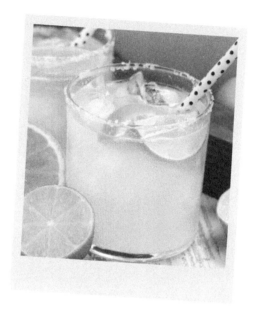

Herbal Fertility Tea

You can buy premade fertility teas online and in brick-and-mortar stores, but making one yourself can be rewarding, cheaper, and repeatable. Once you've found a tea recipe that works for you, start making it in larger batches. Everyone can enjoy this recipe, not just those on a fertility diet.

Time: 10 minutes

Serving Size: 4

Prep Time: 5 minutes

Cook Time: 5 minutes

Nutritional Facts/Info: 4 calories, 0 g fats, 0 g protein, 1 g carbohydrates, 0 g sugar

Ingredients:

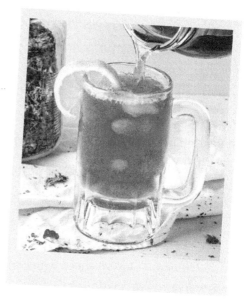

- ½ gallon water
- 4 green tea bags
- 1 bunch red raspberry leaves
- 1 bunch mint leaves
- 2 tbsp lemon juice
- 1 bunch nettle leaves

Directions:

1. Place the red raspberry leaves, mint leaves, and nettle leaves into the bottom of a pitcher and gently muddle them.
2. Using a kettle, bring half a gallon of water to a boil. Pour the boiling water into the pitcher.
3. To the pitcher add four bags of plain green tea and the lemon juice.
4. Allow to steep for ten minutes.
5. Pour and enjoy, reheating as necessary.

Conclusion

When the dishes are done and the stove is cool, you can feel accomplished knowing that you created a delicious dish that also boosts your fertility.

Throughout this guide, you have learned the basics about reproductive health and fertility diets. This process included ingredient lists and shopping guides. We covered the basic diseases that can affect fertility and the other natural ways to combat these ailments, like exercise and supplements. Don't forget to take your vitamins! From the basics, you moved onto crafting delicious dishes for breakfast, lunch, dinner, and dessert. Plus, you got ideas for sides, snacks, and beverages. These meals relied heavily on central ingredients like spinach, pumpkin, chickpeas, oysters, and liver. Some of them even included dietary supplements and powders that can elevate an already fertility friendly meal to the next level. Anytime you can pack in the extra nutrition, make sure to take advantage of the opportunity.

Before getting too excited, and taking a dozen pregnancy tests after your first beef liver taco, remember that it can take up to three months to see any reproductive results based on a dietary lifestyle change. The fertility diet is incredibly effective for those who have patience to see the results.

Also remember to always check with your physician or OB GYN before beginning any new diets. Your doctor will have insights into your specific situation that may be generalized in this or any other book. Keep allergies in mind, and swap ingredients as necessary for allergies or intolerances. The fertility diet can work easily with a gluten free, lactose free, vegetarian or sugar free diet.

If the recipes in this book are successful, then congratulations, you have gone the extra mile to fuel yourself with fertility boosting and hormone balancing foods and hopefully it has paid off. I hope that in no time at all, you have a new, healthy family member sitting at the dining room table. Who knows, maybe some of these recipes will become such a family classic that you will be eating them as a family for years to come.

Key Takeaway Food List

Before you close the book, we want to remind you of the key fertility boosting foods one last time. Take a picture of it, write it down, hang it in the kitchen for all to see, but no matter what you do, refer to this list at all times when experimenting in the kitchen. It is vast across the food pyramid, so you can easily incorporate a fertility friendly ingredient into all your favorite meals, snacks, and drinks. Remember that these foods are beneficial to men and women, and that the fertility diet not only helps you conceive, but it will strengthen the fetus as it grows as well.

- Steak
- Liver
- Salmon
- Eggs
- Sardines
- Pork Belly
- Butter
- Full Fat Dairy
- Whole Milk
- Whole Fat Yogurt
- Cheese
- Asparagus
- Leafy Greens
- Spinach
- Kale
- Pomegranates
- Walnuts
- Brazil Nuts
- Beans
- Pumpkin

- Sweet Potato
- Chickpeas
- Sunflower Seeds
- Citrus Fruits
- Oranges
- Lemon
- Grapefruit
- Cooked Tomatoes
- Avocado
- Oysters
- Cinnamon
- Beets
- Onions

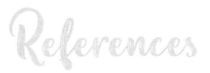

References

4-ingredient watermelon sorbet. (n.d.). Taste of Home. https://www.tasteofhome.com/recipes/4-ingredient-watermelon-sorbet/

10 best teas for fertility to help you get pregnant faster (Reviews). (2021, January 23). Bright Color Mom. https://brightcolormom.com/best-teas-for-fertility/

17 natural ways to boost fertility. (2020, August 13). Healthline. https://www.healthline.com/nutrition/16-fertility-tips-to-get-pregnant

Abraham, L. (2018, April 18). *There's no need for tortillas with taco stuffed avocados*. Delish. https://www.delish.com/cooking/recipe-ideas/a19701670/taco-stuffed-avocados-recipe/

admin. (n.d.). *Baby makin' brownies—Antioxidant-rich bean brownie to boost fertility*. Dr Stefanie Trowell ND | Toronto's Fertility & Women's Health Naturopath. http://nourishtoronto.com/recipe/baby-makin-brownies/

Ali. (2019, February 7). *The best hummus recipe!* Gimme Some Oven. https://www.gimmesomeoven.com/classic-hummus/

Campos, S. (2020, April 3). *Fertility cake*. Sep Cooks. https://sepcooks.com/fertility-cake/

Crazy, B. B. (2016, January 12). *No bake peanut butter protein bites*. Blessed Beyond Crazy. https://blessedbeyondcrazy.com/no-bake-peanut-butter-protein-bites/

Deze. (2021, August 13). *9 effective (& tasty) fertility smoothie recipes for ttc*. ByDeze. https://bydeze.com/best-fertility-smoothie-recipes/

Endometriosis—Symptoms and causes. (n.d.). Mayo Clinic. https://www.mayoclinic.org/diseases-conditions/endometriosis/symptoms-causes/syc-20354656

FertileFoods. (2020, September 22). *Fertility chili recipe to increase fertility and IVF success*. Foods for Fertility. https://foodsforfertility.com/fertility-chili-recipe-to-increase-fertility-and-ivf-success/

Fertility, C. N. Y. (2021, December 15). *The fertility diet—Foods to eat (and avoid) when trying to get pregnant*. CNY Fertility. https://www.cnyfertility.com/fertility-diet/

Fleek, M. P. on. (2018, February 4). *Vegan dark chocolate cinnamon roasted chickpea bark*. Meal Prep on Fleek. https://mealpreponfleek.com/vegan-dark-chocolate-cinnamon-roasted-chickpea-bark/

Kaufman, C. (2020, April 12). *Foods that can affect fertility*. Eat Right. https://www.eatright.org/health/pregnancy/fertility-and-reproduction/fertility-foods

Fried sardines with parsley caper sauce | Italian food forever. (2014, September 9). Italian Food Forever. https://www.italianfoodforever.com/2014/09/fried-sardines-with-parsley-caper-sauce/

Grain-free blueberry muffins | recipe | mymindbodybaby. (n.d.). My Mind Body Baby. https://mymindbodybaby.com/recipes/grain-free-blueberry-muffins/

Grilled beef liver (Keto, paleo, low-carb). (2021, September 5). Yang's Nourishing Kitchen. https://www.yangsnourishingkitchen.com/grilled-beef-liver-kabob/

Gut-friendly roasted pumpkin + forbidden rice holiday salad w/ maple tahini dressing. (2020, November 24). So Fresh N So Green. https://sofreshnsogreen.com/recipes/roasted-pumpkin-holiday-salad/

Have a healthy holiday with these no-bake, paleo sweet potato cheesecake bars. (2019, November 21). So Fresh N So Green. https://sofreshnsogreen.com/recipes/

paleo-cheesecake-bars/

Heidi. (2019, July 19). *Citrus shrimp salad with avocado | foodiecrush.com*. Foodiecrush. https://www.foodiecrush.com/citrus-shrimp-avocado-salad/

Florence, T. (n.d.). *Hollandaise sauce*. Food Network. https://www.foodnetwork.com/recipes/tyler-florence/hollandaise-sauce-recipe-1910043

Hormone balancing Buddha bowl. (2020, October 6). Fertility Help Hub. https://www.fertilityhelphub.com/blog/wellbeing/foods-help-fertility/

jeshaka. (n.d.). *Vegan black bean burgers*. Allrecipes. https://www.allrecipes.com/recipe/222247/vegan-black-bean-burgers/

Joyfulhealthyeats. (2020, January 15). *Easy garlic butter baked salmon in foil—Ready in only 20 min!* Joyful Healthy Eats. https://www.joyfulhealthyeats.com/easy-20-minute-garlic-butter-baked-salmon-in-foil/

Keenan, T. (2008, December). *Sunflower-seed brittle recipe*. Food & Wine. https://www.foodandwine.com/recipes/sunflower-seed-brittle

Littley, C. D. (2019, December 26). *Garlic oysters—A restaurant classic*. Chef Dennis. https://www.askchefdennis.com/garlic-oysters/

Loveless, S. E. (2019, November). *Feta & roasted red pepper stuffed chicken breasts*. EatingWell. https://www.eatingwell.com/recipe/277510/feta-roasted-red-pepper-stuffed-chicken-breasts/

Mixed berry hormone balancing smoothie for ovulation support. (2020, May 25). Traditional Cooking School by GNOWFGLINS. https://traditionalcookingschool.com/food-preparation/mixed-berry-hormone-balancing-smoothie-for-ovulation/?utm_campaign=autoblog&utm_source=blog&utm_medium=bloglink&utm_content=Mixed+Berry+Hormone+Balancing+Smoothie+For+Ovulation+Support

Natalie. (2020, September 17). *Goji berry smoothie*. Natalie's Health. https://www.natalieshealth.com/goji-berry-smoothie/

One bite and your search for the perfect oatmeal raisin cookie is over. (n.d.). Simply Recipes. https://www.simplyrecipes.com/recipes/oatmeal_raisin_cookies/

Oyster stew recipe. (2021, November 12). Chili Pepper Madness. https://www.chilipeppermadness.com/recipes/oyster-stew/

Perry, L. (2019, October 10). *One pot pumpkin curry*. Darn Good Veggies. https://www.darngoodveggies.com/one-pot-pumpkin-curry/

Polycystic ovary syndrome (Pcos)—Symptoms and causes. (n.d.). Mayo Clinic. https://www.mayoclinic.org/diseases-conditions/pcos/symptoms-causes/syc-20353439

Rahne, C. (2022, January 30). *Best homemade cinnamon rolls*. Simply Recipes. https://www.simplyrecipes.com/recipes/bakery_style_cinnamon_rolls/

Rainford, D. (2021, February 13). *Honey garlic roast pork belly slices.* Savvy Bites. https://savvybites.co.uk/honey-garlic-roast-pork-belly-slices/

Sam. (2019, January 30). *The best cheesecake recipe*. Sugar Spun Run. https://sugarspunrun.com/best-cheesecake-recipe/

Sweet potato quinoa bowl. (2015, November 16). Love and Lemons. https://www.loveandlemons.com/quinoa-bowl-recipe/

These 6 foods and nutrients can benefit fertility - blog | everlywell: Home health testing made easy. (n.d.). Everly Well. https://www.everlywell.com/blog/womens-fertility/6-foods-and-nutrients-that-can-boost-a-womans-fertility/

Tuscan white bean stew. (n.d.). Mayo Clinic. https://www.mayoclinic.org/healthy-lifestyle/recipes/tuscan-white-bean-stew/rcp-20049889

Virgin mojito (Non-alcoholic mojito mocktail). (2021, April 12). 40 Aprons. https://40aprons.com/virgin-mojito/

What you need to know about your fertility. (2017, July 9). Cedars-Sinai. https://www.cedars-sinai.org/blog/need-know-fertility.html

Why am I not getting pregnant? (n.d.). NoMoNauseaBand. https://nomonausea.com/blogs/healthandwellness/why-cant-i-get-pregnant

Your new healthy fall snack hack is here—Easy pumpkin hummus (Vegan/gluten-free). (2019, October 23). So Fresh N So Green. https://sofreshnsogreen.com/recipes/your-new-healthy-fall-snack-hack-is-here-easy-pumpkin-hummus-vegan-gluten-free/

Made in the USA
Las Vegas, NV
11 October 2024

96664107R00131